The Sitting Disease

Restore Your Posture and Eliminate
Body Pain in 10 Minutes a Day

Dr. Heidi Roberts, PT, DPT
with Katie Roberts
ILLUSTRATIONS BY JULIE ROCHA BUEL

Reader Resources

Head over to **motiontherapy.net** to explore materials that will help you integrate pain-free posture tools, techniques, and strategies into your life. Start living with greater energy and confidence today!

Follow Motion Therapy

Website: www.motiontherapy.net
Facebook: www.facebook.com/MotionTherapyPT
Instagram: www.instagram.com/motiontherapypt
Twitter: www.twitter.com/MotionTherapyPT

Written by Katie Roberts
Book illustrations by Julie Rocha Buel
Book design by Jennifer Stimson
Edited by Christina Roth
Author Photo by Jen Jones
Publishing Services by Paper Raven Books

Paperback ISBN = 978-0-692-93557-6
Hardback ISBN = 978-0-692-93116-5

To Tim—I love you.

Contents

Preface

"The greatest medicine of all is teaching people how not to need it."

—HIPPOCRATES

There's no escaping it. Chronic pain due to postural imbalance, repetitive-use injuries, and a sedentary lifestyle is one of the most costly and debilitating challenges facing society today.

Why? The human body didn't evolve for the purpose of a sedentary lifestyle. Our bodies are designed to move. And yet our busy digital and technology-driven lives have created serious problems for ambitious workers, creators, and entrepreneurs. We spend hours a day sitting at our computers, at our desks, and in our cars. We live each day with minimal whole-body movement. We slump over our iPhones, workstations, and dinner tables.

These habits profoundly affect the body, mind, and spirit. Extensive research shows that **Sitting Disease**—or the state of physical, mental, or emotional pain that results from being sedentary—is greatly to blame. You're probably familiar with a number of the symptoms—everything from neck and back pain to depression, obesity, heart disease, and even cancer. A growing and costly problem, Sitting Disease is one of the cornerstones to so many acute and chronic health-care conditions today. In fact, it has become a veritable epidemic in modern-day society.

Responding to this crisis and your own experience with pain, *The Sitting Disease: Restore Your Posture and Eliminate Body Pain in 10 Minutes a Day* brings you a proven solution. Here, you'll find an inspiring, science-based, and practical guide designed to support your health and wellness journey. This guidebook will empower you to move from pain toward possibility through practical, actionable steps.

You will learn how to:

- eliminate pain and prevent injury with a *10-Minute Body Maintenance System*.
- design your life to manage your body imbalances and set goals to live pain-free.
- accelerate your productivity and enhance performance with powerful habits.

You will gain:

1. Time for yourself, family, and interests without nagging aches and pains chipping away at your life.
2. Money to invest, spend, or give away by being proactive with your health rather than reactive.
3. Energy in the activities that you can perform without pain, imbalance, or injury.
4. Feelings of ease—physically, mentally, and emotionally—along with clarity and confidence to sustain gains you make by regularly applying this guidebook's Tools & Techniques.
5. Increased productivity and performance because you will overcome roadblocks and will be equipped with a system to prevent pain and injury.

This guidebook helps you determine how you *truly* want to feel in your body. It gives you knowledge, practical techniques and tools, and the system to achieve your goals. Whether you're stuck at a desk job or are already moving about your life in a fairly regular way, let me meet you where you are in your day-to-day life. Here I offer you a specific and strategic system that can be integrated into your busy life to inspire action, drive change, and help you live pain-free, energized, and confident.

Introduction

> "A body in motion tends to stay in motion unless acted upon by an outside force."
>
> **—ISAAC NEWTON**

I n the twenty-first century, we're all aware of the dangers of smoking and a diet of only fast food and sugary soda. But you might have noticed a number of headlines exposing some rather shocking yet science- and research-based studies over the past few years. What they're telling us: the dangers of a sedentary lifestyle are real.

"Sitting Is the New Smoking—Even for Runners," declared *Runner's World* magazine.[1]

"Get Up. Get Out. Don't Sit," wrote the *New York Times*.[2]
And "Don't Just Sit There. Really," declared the *Los Angeles Times*.[3]

The truth had hit mainstream media in a paramount way. Numerous studies were linking excessive sitting to chronic disease, sickness, and pain. And the trending stories adequately captured what I had repeatedly witnessed in my own profession. Here are the facts:

Sitting Too Much . . .

· IS DEADLY.

Approximately 36 percent of adults in the United States do not engage in any physical activity in their free time. Lack of physical activity accounts for 22 percent of coronary heart disease, 22 percent of colon cancer, 18 percent of osteoporotic fractures, 12 percent of diabetes and hypertension, and 5 percent of breast cancer.
—*Science Daily*[4]

• COSTS A LOT.

At least 100 million Americans live with chronic pain, with the resulting treatments and productivity loss costing an estimated $635 billion. —*Harvard*[5]

• IMPACTS OUR ABILITY TO WORK.

In the United States, 7.6 million people list back/spine pain as their reason for filing disability claims. It's the second most common reason for filing these claims. —*Centers for Disease Control and Prevention*[6]

• COMPROMISES THE BOTTOM LINE.

Worker illness and injury costs United States employers $225.8 billion annually. —*Centers for Disease Control Foundation*[7]

• MAKES US SICK.

Too much sitting is linked to serious disease and premature death. —*Harvard Health Publications*[8]

• IS THE "NEW SMOKING."

Every hour of television watched may reduce our life span by an average of 21.8 minutes. Smoking a cigarette, on the other hand, reduces our life span by about 11 minutes. —*British Journal of Sports Medicine*[9]

An Active Lifestyle . . .

• RESOLVES PAIN.

Sit-to-stand workstations that reduced sitting by a mere 66 minutes per day reduced upper back and neck pain by 54 percent. Meanwhile, 75 percent of people also felt healthier overall. —*Centers for Disease Control and Prevention*[10]

· IS A PROVEN WEIGHT-LOSS SOLUTION.

A person can lose about 8 pounds per year just by standing an extra three hours per day. —*University of Chester, United Kingdom*[11]

· IS THE ATHLETE'S BEST-KEPT SECRET.

Runners and others in training can better boost strength and wellness by incorporating activity throughout the day. In fact, running an hour every morning will not make up for the damage done by sitting for the other 15 hours or so that you're awake. It's not too little physical activity that hurts our bodies, it's sitting too much. —*Runner's World*[12]

· SUSTAINS HEART HEALTH.

For every hour spent sitting, five minutes of walking is enough to reverse harmful effects caused to arteries in the legs. —*Indiana University*[13]

· IMPROVES PERFORMANCE.

Workers feel 66 percent more productive using standing workstations as opposed to sitting. —*Centers for Disease Control and Prevention*[14]

· ENHANCES A CHILD'S LIFE.

Studies show moving classrooms and standing desks for children increase physical activity, decrease obesity, and improve the odds of preventing future back pain. —*Journal of Public Health (Oxford)*[15]

The solution that *works* is one that gets to the root cause of your symptoms to resolve pain and imbalance. It empowers you to create and sustain an active lifestyle, no matter how busy you are, how old you are, or how fit you are. And it applies to all aspects of what you do and how you feel. The solution is all about guiding you in how you work. How you play. How you create. It's not just about what's ailing you at the moment.

As a doctor of physical therapy, I regularly work with people in pain. Many of these people are probably like you: they consider themselves at least somewhat active—they work out at the gym, run several miles a week, play with their kids or grandkids— yet they come to me struggling with chronic pain from being sedentary most of the day. And they don't know what steps to take to manage their pain, especially those who've tried and failed a number of so-called solutions. I needed to find a practical way to educate and empower others plus hold them accountable where they were: *real time, real life, real world*. What people needed was a strategic solution to build the right **habits**, achieve goals, and remain accountable to ***practice*** along their health and wellness journey.

This guidebook is that solution. I created it through the real-time application of science, testing every step along the way until my clients successfully implemented a system for individual body maintenance. In fact, this specific yet simple system was so successful with my clients that it inspired me to bring these practical techniques, tools, and strategies to you.

There are three parts to this guidebook:

1. Pain & Possibility: reflecting on your pain, creating your powerful vision of what your pain-free life will look like, and establishing goals that support how you want to feel in your body.
2. Tools & Techniques: learning, implementing, and practicing "mindful" movement that empowers your active lifestyle.
3. Results & Outcomes: sustaining your active lifestyle through habits that I call the "3Cs: Commitment, Convenience, and Consistency."

Essentially, this guidebook builds on the concepts and therapies of body motion to offer a practical prescription for anyone who is sedentary at work and wants to address their pain symptoms, body imbalances, or chronic physical conditions. Specifically, you'll design your life to sustain your active lifestyle, using a powerful strategy: the 10-Minute Body Maintenance System. That's right—as little as 10 minutes of body maintenance a day results in a less sedentary and more active lifestyle. The goal: to live pain-free, energized, and confident.

PART I

Pain & Possibility

"We change our behavior when the pain of staying the same becomes greater than the pain of changing. Consequences give us the pain that motivates us to change." — **HENRY CLOUD**

The essence of being alive is movement. Think about it—we're *homo sapiens*. We spent millions of years evolving these complicated feet, strong legs, and subtly curved spines so we can stand upright and move about our lives. We're built to do this. Yet we disregard this fact and take our systems for granted, engaging in constant, chronic sitting.

Americans are sitting an average of 13 hours a day and sleeping an average of 8 hours.[16] This is resulting in a sedentary lifestyle of around 21 hours a day. Yet while American adults know about the importance of exercise, only 31 percent go to the gym, and 56 percent devote less than $10 per month to staying active.

Your life is movement, and your movement defines your life. So think for a moment. What would it feel like to have the flexibility to pick up your child without pain? Or complete your first 5K or half marathon? Perhaps sleep a full night without waking from back pain?

In working with people who want to be healthier and live pain-free, I've found they need knowledge to understand their body, guidance to relieve their pain, and accountability to sustain their

They needed a solution that was effective, efficient, and sustainable. The answer was a *proactive* versus *reactive* approach to health and wellness. Movement was—and remains—the answer.

results. I'm here to guide you on your health and wellness journey so that you, too, can have lasting results. But first, let me share a short story about my own journey.

Fresh out of college, I launched a career in corporate financial management. It wasn't a great fit. Then I moved on to other jobs that also didn't align with my innate purpose, or who I really was and how I needed to move, feel, and simply be. Over time, I developed significant physical pain that manifested as a host of symptoms. I became ill more frequently, developing problems from shingles to pneumonia and even fainting episodes. So I course-corrected and retooled for a career in health and wellness. I was seeking autonomy, knowledge, and the skills to change people's lives, including my own. I learned the amazing intricacies of the human body—and how to listen to my body. With this, I could help myself first and then others on their journey to greater health and wellness.

After graduating and completing my post-doctorate residency, I realized education and empowering others needed to be at the forefront of my work. People deserved to get results, and the only way was to get to the root of their pain. They needed a solution that was effective, efficient, and sustainable. The answer was a *proactive* versus *reactive* approach to health and wellness. Movement was—and remains—the answer.

With more clarity, I adopted a new mindset, created a new business, and practiced and modeled a new way of living. The business, called Motion Therapy, shares solutions with people in pain and rewards them as they make gains toward their pain-free lifestyle. Specifically, it supports those who desire to manage the common imbalances that result from too much time sitting.

Problems from Head to Toe

Don't Just Sit There!

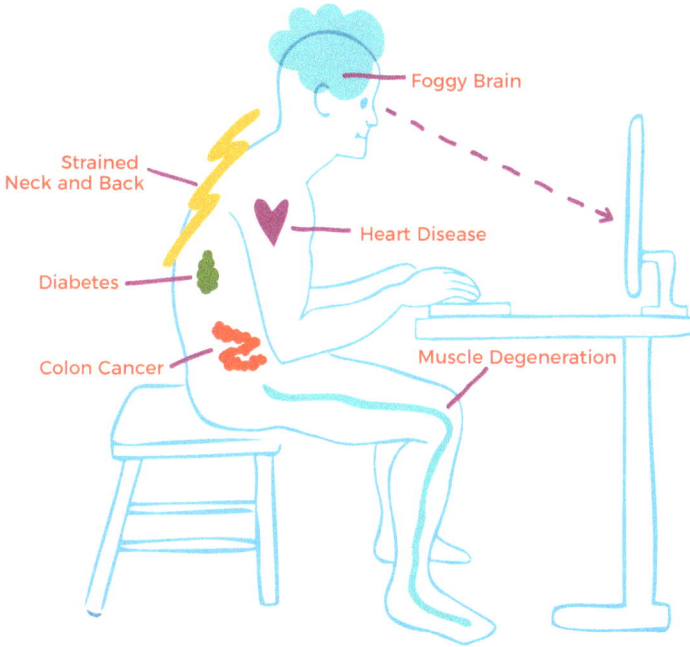

Research indicates it's more movement that we need, not just more standing. Take a look at all the contributing factors from excessive sitting as shown in the illustration on page 3. Movement offsets inadequate respiration, organ damage, muscle degeneration, leg disorders, back and neck strain, and more.

If you're reading this book, something is inviting or driving you to create and sustain your active lifestyle. You're ready for the truth behind the sedentary lifestyle so you can stop feeling depleted and start feeling energized—no matter where you are or what you're doing. You're about to get the proven techniques and tools, and I will be your guide.

Unpack Your Pain

"Trust yourself. Create the kind of self that you will be happy to live with all your life."

—GOLDA MEIR

The cornerstone to your success on your health and wellness journey is understanding both your *pain and possibility*. Many people want a quick fix. I don't blame them—who doesn't want to feel instantly at ease and cured of all aches and pains? I do! Although your success might not be quick, it also doesn't require a complicated or time-consuming solution.

It wasn't too long ago that Amy came to me because of her grabbing low back pain and hip tightness. She is an independent-type business owner in her late thirties, someone who is highly creative and innovative in both her personal and professional life. When she shared her story, it became clear her pain was preventing her from sitting comfortably while driving and working on her laptop.

Amy had seen a number of health-care providers but hadn't completely resolved her symptoms. She was struggling to keep up with her home exercise program. By integrating the 10-Minute Body Maintenance System (chapter 7) into her workday, she learned to hold herself accountable. She did this

> The cornerstone to your success on your health and wellness journey is understanding both your *pain and possibility.*

The pain-free life is not out of your reach. It starts by understanding where you've been and getting a good idea of where you are going.

through making the system a habit and continuing daily to practice her stretches and exercises. She went from the hassle of seeing a whole of host of providers (all with different ideas of what she should do) to not needing anyone except herself. And truth is, I loved that she eventually became pain-free. My goal with all my clients is for them to not need me. What this means is the solution works. And it does.

Steven regularly travels internationally and found that his neck and mid back bothered him on flights, commutes, and long days in the office. He was frustrated with the temporary fixes and the ongoing time and effort it was taking. By gaining knowledge about regular movement and proper alignment, he discovered the "why" behind his pain and how to prevent his problems, reduce risk, and integrate the critical motion he needed into his life. Once he had this knowledge and took action, he changed the behavior that was causing his pain in the first place. Today, he lives pain-free.

The pain-free life is not out of your reach. It starts by understanding where you've been and getting a good idea of where you are going, using the very same tools and techniques as both Amy and Steven. Let's get started.

How would you describe your current condition? Think about what's going on with your body. Is there tightness in your upper back and neck? Numbness and tingling in your left hand? Or low back pain?

Whatever is going on, it's important to put adjectives to what you're feeling. Describe the particular sensation and where it is located. Think about the factors that aggravate and ease your symptoms.

Name your condition, symptoms, or pain here, using those specific adjectives. For example, is it sharp, dull, throbbing, numbing, stinging, intermittent, or constant?

My current condition:

Where I feel it:

How it feels:

Rate your symptoms on a scale of 1 to 10 (1 = no pain, 10 = extreme pain):

1   2   3   4   5   6   7   8   9   10

I notice my symptoms increase and decrease when I am doing this activity:

What are your functional limitations? Think about how your pain, condition, or symptoms prevent you from doing day-to-day activities. Perhaps you cannot lift your left arm above your head, or turning your head while driving feels impossible. Or maybe when you're running, you can't go as far as you'd like before knee pain stops you. What are your functional limitations? What activities feel impossible?

My body's movement is restricted in these areas:

What's the progression of your condition? Dive a little deeper, going back into your past. Try to remember when the pain started or when the story of the pain began. Also, think about times in which the condition, pain, or symptoms changed, improved, or worsened. What was going on? What were you doing differently? What, if any, major events were or are still taking place in your life?

For example, maybe your low back pain began after an injury 20 years ago but increased after starting a new job. Since that new situation, it's only gotten worse year after year. Or maybe you bought that new office chair and noticed the low back pain annoys you more as the day goes on.

Sometimes the story of our condition doesn't make sense until we think about the plot and connect the dots. Notice repeating patterns or when trigger events have contributed to the progression of your pain. Your story may be short and sweet or more complicated. Either way, move it out of your head onto the pages of this guidebook. Powerful insights will appear when we connect what is in our head to what is in our hearts and bodies.

Spend some time thinking about whether the pain had a date of onset, and consider any incidents, surgeries, injuries, or other possible key changes in your life.

My condition has a story. It goes like this:

Physical Body Scan

If you're feeling a little stuck with what to write about your story or simply want to learn a really powerful assessment tool for identifying pain, do a quick **body scan**.

Right where you are, whether sitting or standing, be still for a minute or two. Notice and ask:

What am I feeling?
Where am I feeling it?
How would I rate the pain, such as on a scale of 1 to 10?

This technique takes just a few minutes but can be very powerful. It offers self-awareness, and this leads to insight. From new insights about your body, you gain clarity and will notice imbalances in your body. Once you've got this information, you'll get clues on the next steps to take.

Before we get to any specific techniques or exercises to manage your pain, let's look at why you *really* want to live pain-free.

2

Know How You Want to Feel

"Knowing how you actually want to feel is the most potent form of clarity that you can have. Generating those feelings is the most powerfully creative thing you can do with your life."

—DANIELLE LAPORTE, THE DESIRE MAP

There are a few really important questions that I ask clients when we are creating their health and wellness plan. One question is, "What is your vision?" If they don't have a **vision** of where they want to go, then they really struggle to set goals.

It's essential to have a clear vision of the big, broad goal in your life—where you ultimately want to go. You need to be able to see this destination in your mind's eye and have a vivid understanding of what that vision looks like, physically and mentally. But equally important, you must determine how this vision makes you feel.

My client Ben lives and breathes adventure travel and has designed his business to enable independence of location. He wants to be fit and ready to go on any adventure that life brings his way. His vision was simple: to be injury-free, strong, and confident, in spite of long days running his business, so he can be prepared when an opportunity comes his way.

What's your vision?

Your vision is what you're going to keep in mind as you work daily to achieve it. When you're faced with indecision, doubt, or fear around whatever goal you're setting, you can return to that vision and ask whether what you're doing aligns with it. If it doesn't, then that goal won't get you where you need to go.

Your vision gives you a basis for this handy litmus test. It determines why you need to do—or not do—what you're doing. Your vision is that motivating and inspiring destination you've purposely crafted. It's the big, broad, exciting picture of your future.

Your vision is *not* something you're just sitting around and hoping will happen. It's tied to goals you set and actions you will take. Remember, this is *your journey*, and it is your *lifelong practice*.

Now that you've written down your vision, next ask:

How do you want to feel in your body?

Good, I'm sure! But defining exactly how you want to feel in your body is going to be the bridge between your pain and possibility.

As Danielle LaPorte describes in one of my favorite books, *The Desire Map*, identifying and describing your core desired feelings is about knowing how you actually want to feel and recognizing the incredible power in creating goals with soul. Understanding how you want to feel is what gives clarity. It's part of a creative process that enables you to discover what you need to actually do in your life.

Your vision is not something you're just sitting around and hoping will happen. It's tied to goals you set and actions you will take.

How do you want to feel in your body? Be specific. Do you want to feel confident? Vibrant? Beautiful? Stable? Flexible? Strong? Energized? Invincible? Lean? Light? Pain-free? Informed? Inspired? Attractive?

Name those core feelings here:

What activities will empower these feelings?

Incorporating routine body maintenance habits is critical to achieving your desired feelings— and ultimately your vision.

When we can't function normally or do activities we love without pain, we experience internal and external limitations. When we hurt, it can be hard to participate in sports with our kids, for example. Or if we're in enough pain, it can actually steal our total independence, requiring us to rely on someone to help us get dressed or go to the bathroom.

Don't dwell on these limitations. There are no judgments here. Rather, identify what you would like to be able to do to feel your "core desired feelings."

For example, like many parents, Jill was a busy mom who wanted to lose 10 pounds. She juggled competing priorities of managing the household, building her online business, and losing the baby weight. She wanted to experience freedom in her body. She wanted to feel light, beautiful, and energized. Renewed.

Intentionally choosing *daily activities* that made Jill feel light, beautiful, and energized ignited some powerful changes. She went to yoga. She started a walking program. And she implemented the 10-Minute Body Maintenance System as part of her lunchtime routine. Incorporating routine body maintenance habits, like Jill did, is critical to achieving your desired feelings—and ultimately your vision.

Here, commit to implementing routine body maintenance habits that will actually support your feeling the way you want to feel. If there are many activities, start with the three that feel most critical for you today.

The activities I'd like to perform:

Remember, what you uniquely desire to feel is what ultimately inspires you. It's the key motivator, what will empower you to create body maintenance habits, achieve your goals, and make progress toward living your vision.

3

Use Your Vision to Create Your Goals

"It doesn't matter if it takes a long time getting there; the point is to have a destination."

—EUDORA WELTY

Before taking the next step, it's essential to talk about your *goals*. Goals are practical, attainable outcomes that you plan for and believe move you toward your vision. More than mere hopes or wishes, they are concrete stepping-stones that lead you down the path of a valued life. They get you closer and closer to your vision with each success.

Short-term goals equate to small successes that create momentum as you achieve them.

Goals are waypoints in your roadmap, places you plan to visit as you move toward your ultimate destination. And your goals should always align with your vision. To move away from a state of pain and toward your possibility, you will need both **long-term goals** and **short-term goals**.

Short-term goals equate to small successes that create momentum as you achieve them. For instance, if you've had a major knee surgery, your short-term goals may be getting out of bed independently, using the restroom unassisted, and walking

Long-term goals become your ultimate reality. about the room. If you're experiencing back pain at your desk, maybe set a timer to remind you to stand up and stretch on the hour, every hour, for 10 minutes.

Long-term goals become your ultimate reality. They may include incorporating the 10-Minute Body Maintenance System into your day, eventually making it part of your lifestyle. Or they may include ditching the desk and creating an active workstation instead (see Chapter 6). As you accomplish each long-term goal, it simply comes to be part of your life.

Write Down Your SMART Goals

Whenever setting goals, whether short-term or long-term, follow these two important rules. First, whatever goals you set, get them down on paper. The most important determinant of a goal's success is writing it down. Second, make sure the goals are **SMART goals**: those that are Specific, Measurable, Attainable, Realistic, and Time-bound.

Specific: Moving more is not specific. Standing is more specific. Standing at your workstation is even more specific.

Measurable: You must be able to track whether you have met your goal. For example, "I will stand three more hours a day" is something you can track daily. The success of it (or lack thereof) becomes measurable.

Attainable: "I will stand every day for five hours a day" might be shooting for the stars at first for some people. To keep it attainable, consider: "I will stand 30 minutes every hour between 9 a.m. and 3 p.m."

Realistic: Make sure the goal fits into your life right now and is something you really want to do. Establishing new habits may

A SMART goal is one that's . . .

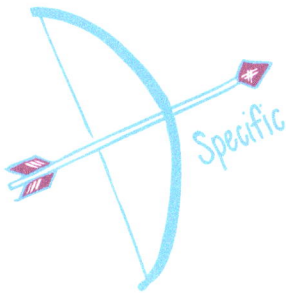

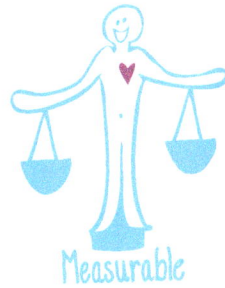

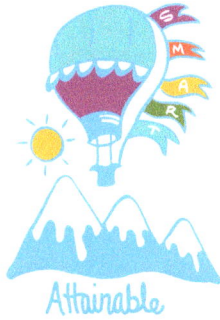

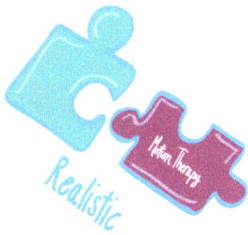

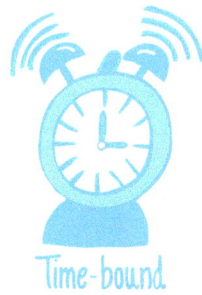

be tough during a major life event. For example, starting an aggressive exercise routine when you're 28 weeks pregnant is likely not realistic.

Time-bound: Give your goal an end point so you can then measure and check its success. At that point, you may want to reset the goal or extend that time frame, but a goal that has no end date will yield poor results and loss of momentum.

With these guidelines in mind:

"I'm going to get up and move more" is not a SMART goal.

"I'm going to stand at my workstation for three additional hours per day, five days per week, over the next two weeks" is a SMART goal.

Write your short-term health and wellness goals here:

Write your long-term health and wellness goals here:

Now, check these goals against how you want to feel and your vision. Do these objectives support your vision? Do the goals you listed have potential to deliver the feelings you desire? If so, I'm willing to bet you've chosen the best goals for you in *your time, your life, your real world.*

Keep these goals in mind as you move on to Part II, where you'll be taking action by implementing the system, tools, and techniques that will support you on your health and wellness journey.

PART II

Tools & Techniques

f you are feeling a bit overwhelmed after reading through Part I and doing the various exercises, I want you to know that this feeling is okay—it's normal. In fact, it's a good sign you have discovered some core truths about your vision, desired feelings in your body, and SMART goals.

Trust in yourself. And then let's move forward with what's undeniably the heart of this guide: the techniques, tools, and strategies that will show you step-by-step how to transform your pain into the realization of your possibility while you work. On the following page is your Roadmap to Recovery that will help you visualize that transformation.

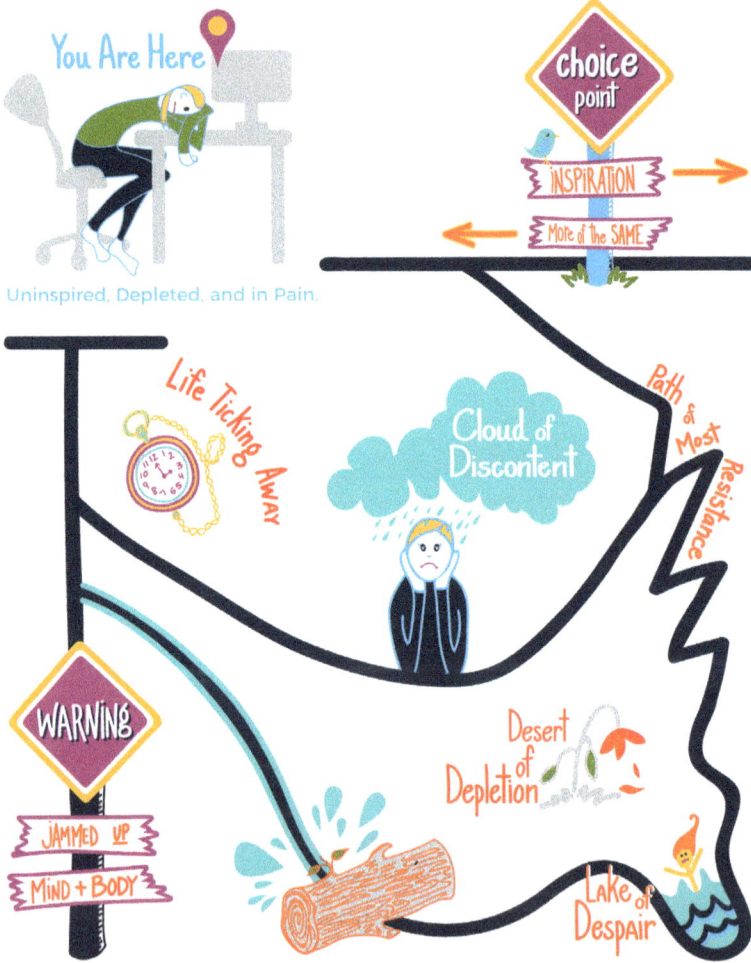

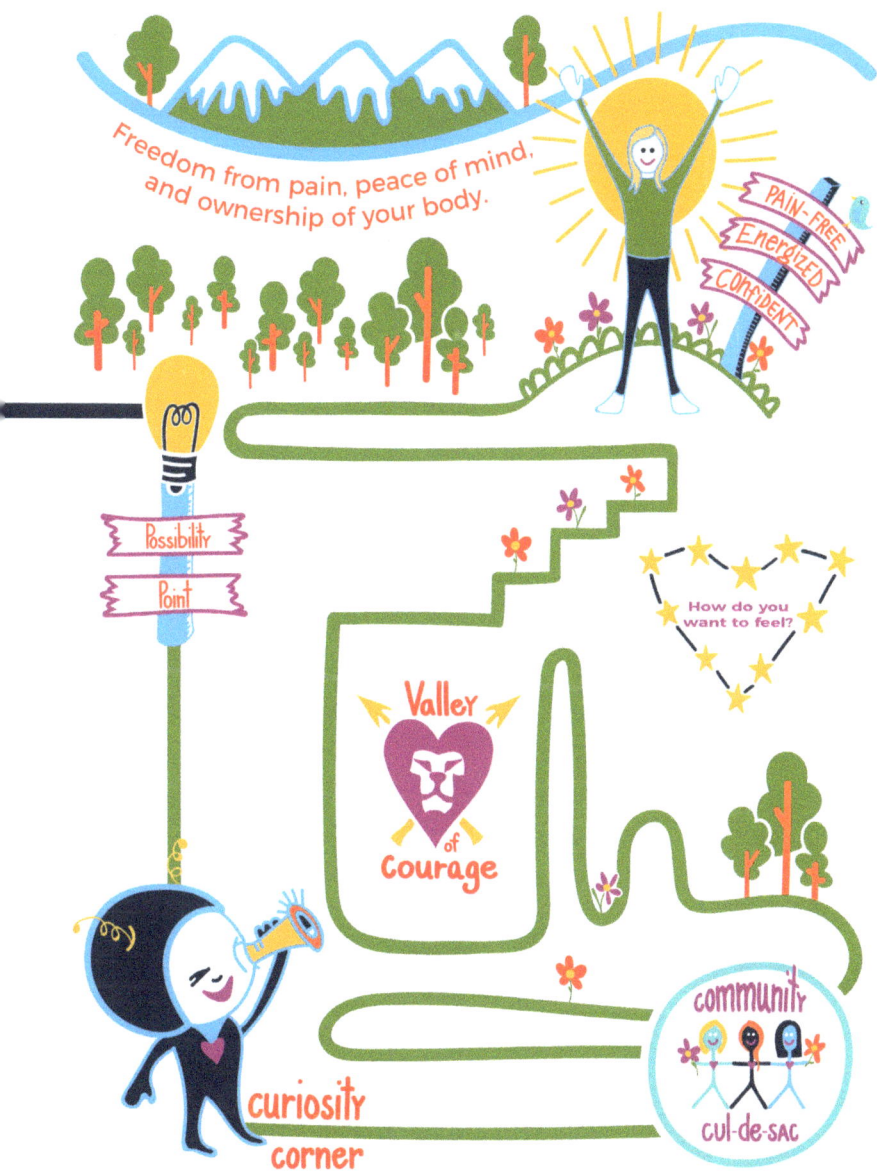

Freedom from pain, peace of mind, and ownership of your body.

PAIN-FREE

Energized

CONFIDENT

Possibility Point

How do you want to feel?

Valley of Courage

curiosity corner

community cul-de-sac

Here in Part II, you'll learn how to prevent and eliminate the pain from too much sitting by learning, applying, and practicing:

- Techniques: Posture & Alignment to Invite "Shift"
- Tools: Active Workstation Design & Body Maintenance Tools
- Strategy: the 10-Minute Body Maintenance System

These techniques, tools, and strategies set the foundation for living and sustaining an active lifestyle that will enable you to live pain-free.

4

Posture, Alignment, & the Root Cause of Your Pain

"It is through the alignment of the body that I discovered the alignment of my mind, self, and intelligence."

—B.K.S. IYENGAR

The Root Cause of Your Pain

I n working with clients, I've found that the most common, troublesome, and painful imbalances in the body result from a sedentary lifestyle. As stated earlier, Sitting Disease consists of symptoms that result from a sedentary lifestyle (too much time at the desk job, on the computer, in the chair, etc.). What many people don't realize is why excessive sitting leads to aches and pains from head to toe and the common imbalances at the root of their pain. It all comes down to poor posture.

Posture plays an important role in how we live, work, and play. In fact, I've educated my clients about the problems, solutions, and rewards related to proper posture more than any other topic.

Posture

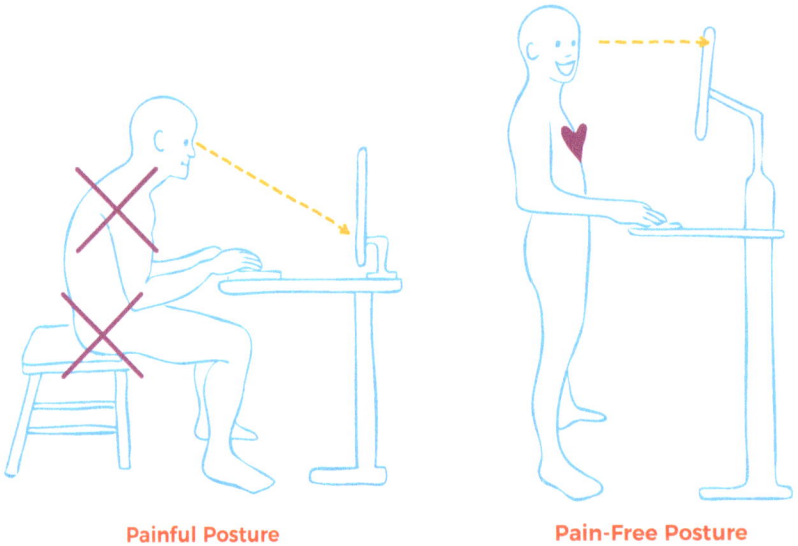

Painful Posture   Pain-Free Posture

Alignment is about what's connected. Posture is about what's seen.

Take a look at the sitting and standing figures in the illustration. "Bad posture" usually comes to mind when most people look at the figure at left, while "good posture" is what most people think of when considering the figure at the right.

Depending on the person, postural imbalances can manifest in many different ways and places within the body. In the next illustration, you can see that poor posture and alignment are the source of the muscular imbalances called **Upper Crossed Syndrome** and **Lower Crossed Syndrome**. Note the X's in this illustration. The X's indicate how the opposing group of tight muscles and weak muscles are the source of imbalance.

Upper + Lower Crossed Syndromes

In Upper Crossed Syndrome, the imbalances are focused in the upper part of the body, mostly the neck, shoulders, upper back, and chest.

When the upper trapezius and pectoral muscles get too tight and the cervical flexors and lower traps get too weak, these imbalances perpetuate a forward head, rounded shoulders and a hunched upper spine

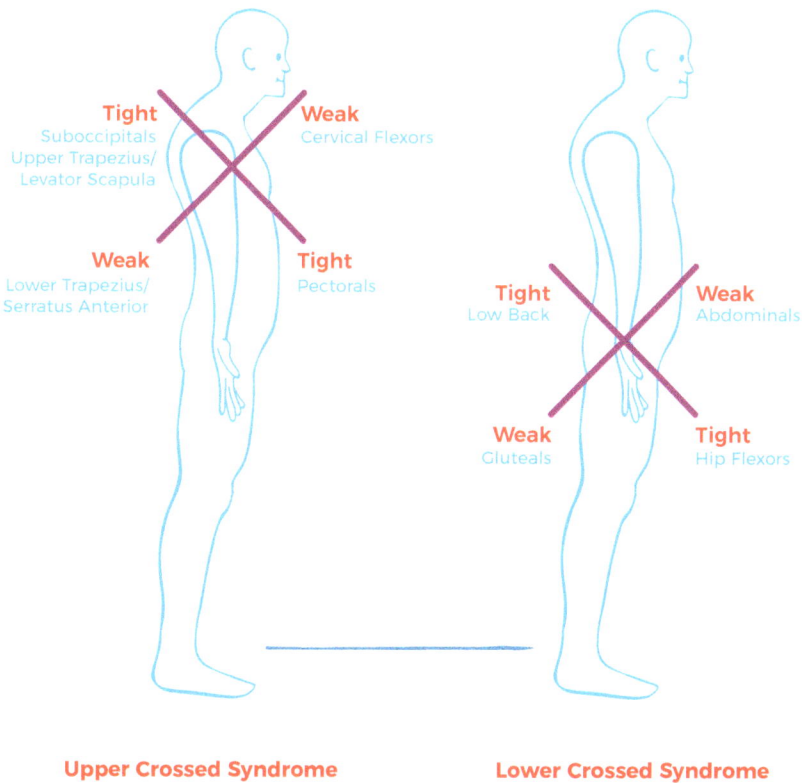

Tight
Suboccipitals
Upper Trapezius/
Levator Scapula

Weak
Cervical Flexors

Weak
Lower Trapezius/
Serratus Anterior

Tight
Pectorals

Tight
Low Back

Weak
Abdominals

Weak
Gluteals

Tight
Hip Flexors

Upper Crossed Syndrome   **Lower Crossed Syndrome**

In Lower Crossed Syndrome, the imbalances are centered on the pelvis, low back, hip, and abdominal region.

When the low back and hip muscles get too tight and glutes and abs get too weak, these imbalances perpetuate a forward belly, inwardly curved lower spine, and jammed-up hips.

These imbalances result from too much sitting, leading to muscle dysfunction, pain, and injury.

Proper Posture Reflects Proper Alignment

So, why does proper posture really matter? Proper posture is an outward sign that your body is accurately aligned. Accurate *alignment* of the body is *the way* to set all other wheels in motion. When all 640 muscles and 206 bones are in optimal alignment, your "system" is primed for optimal performance, and you can perform activities efficiently, effectively, and without pain or limitation. It's simply how our bodies are designed.

Remember, *alignment is about what's connected. Posture is about what's seen.*

Alignment is dynamic. When your body aligns as it is designed to do, you will move through your day with confidence and peace of mind. You will activate the very same muscles that people strive to perfect by spending countless hours at the gym and thousands of dollars for "core training."

Posture is static. It's essentially a snapshot of how you hold your body at any given moment. And since you are a breathing, living, human being on the move, your posture is constantly changing. Thus, we are

Regardless of whether you're standing or sitting, your goal should be optimal alignment. That's a huge factor in managing the imbalances and eliminating resulting pain symptoms of Upper and Lower Crossed Syndromes.

focusing on "alignment" rather than "posture" as you transform your life through a dynamic and active lifestyle at home, work, and play.

Regardless of whether you're standing or sitting, your goal should be optimal alignment. That's a huge factor in managing the imbalances and eliminating resulting pain symptoms of Upper and Lower Crossed Syndromes.

Now that you've learned the importance of proper alignment as you move through your day, it's time to turn your focus inward, specifically looking at how your breath facilitates healthy natural alignment and movement at the core of your body.

5

Breath, Mindful Building of Your Core

"The important thing is not to stop questioning. Curiosity has its own reason for existing."

—EINSTEIN

A s we discussed earlier, Sitting Disease eventually leads to varying degrees of whole-body dysfunction. Ultimately, it can be disabling to the body, mind, and spirit. However, it's totally preventable and often reversible for millions of people just like you. How?

You start by building awareness, knowledge, and self-initiative, specifically by getting curious about your sitting habits. A great way to do this is to spend at least one day tracking the amount of time you are seated. These "Sitting Stats" will provide a snapshot of the approximate number of hours you're sitting in a static posture versus leading an active, more dynamic lifestyle. With this powerful tool, you'll achieve a greater awareness of your sedentary behaviors. You'll also better understand your risk for developing Sitting Disease.

In reviewing your "Sitting Stats," don't be too surprised if you've found you're sitting a lot. "More than half of the average person's waking hours are spent sitting: watching television, working at a computer, commuting, or doing other physically inactive pursuits."[17] Chronic sitting is the biggest reason why so many people are experiencing unnecessary pain and why I created this guidebook to help.

My Sitting Stats

It is powerful to assess how much time we sit in our day-to-day life. Use this self-assessment tool to keep track of your sedentary hours in one 24-hour period.

Eat Breakfast	_____ Hours
Commute to Work	_____ Hours
Work in the Morning	_____ Hours
Eat Lunch	_____ Hours
Work in the Afternoon	_____ Hours
Commute Home	_____ Hours
Eat Dinner	_____ Hours
Relax/Leisure	_____ Hours
Sleep	_____ Hours
Total Sedentary Time:	_____ Hours

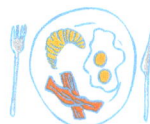

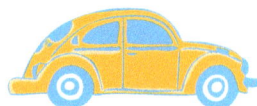

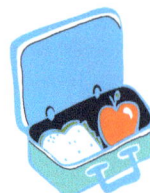

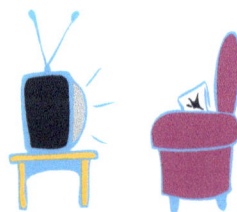

In addition to chronic sitting, many of us have also unconsciously picked up another habit: shallow, restricted breathing developed because of poor posture when sitting. With shallow breathing, fresh oxygenated air tends to circulate only within the upper chest as opposed to deep in the belly with purposeful diaphragmatic breathing.

Without purposeful and deep breathing, core muscles weaken. And as mentioned earlier, when the core is weak from chronic sitting and poor posture, you're more likely to develop Upper or Lower Crossed Syndrome.

Breath is one of the most powerful, oft-overlooked tools we have in our toolbox for pain-free living. Just as moving is *living*, breath is *life*, and giving your body more of the life it needs can relieve stress and anxiety, facilitate healthy digestion, build immunity, provide physical comfort, and enhance overall well-being. Proactively engaging your breathing muscles in a natural, balanced way—that is, with **mindful breathing**—contributes to good alignment.

Core Muscles

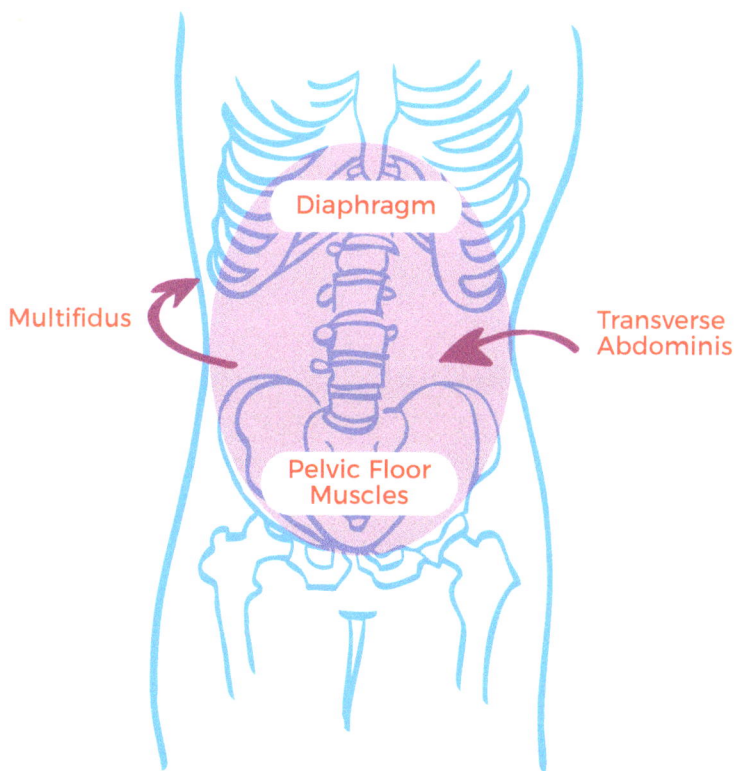

Diaphragm

Multifidus

Transverse Abdominis

Pelvic Floor Muscles

In preparing for our next action steps, take a look at the next two pictures. The first shows how breath connects to the core. The second illustration on balloon breathing outlines how to breathe effectively and strengthen diaphragmatic muscles and the entire core at the same time.[18]

Your Breath + Core

Inhalation: When breathing in, your diaphragm contracts, moving air in and downward.

Exhalation: When breathing out, your diaphragm relaxes, moving air upward and out.

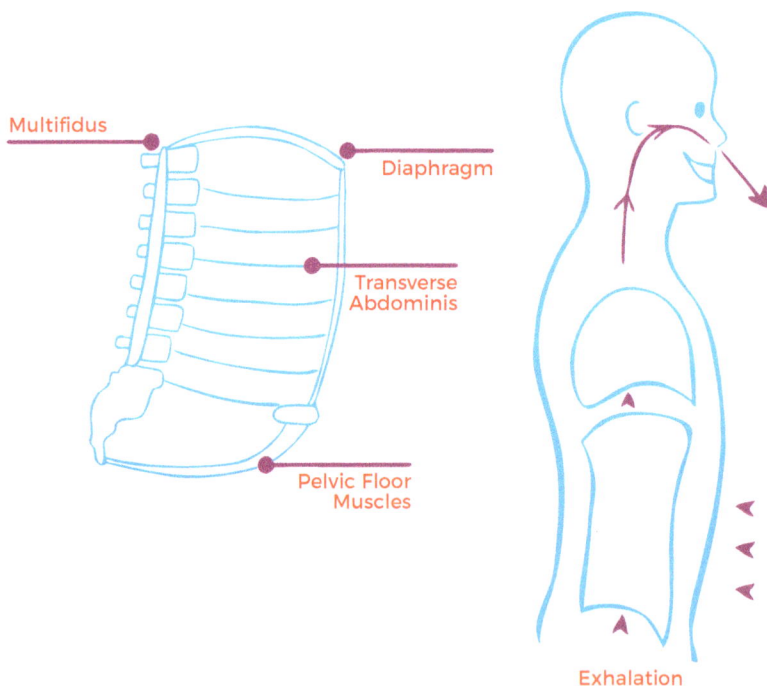

Multifidus

Diaphragm

Transverse Abdominis

Pelvic Floor Muscles

Exhalation

When breathing in (inhaling), your diaphragm contracts, moving oxygenated air in and downward into the chest cavity.

When breathing out (exhaling), your diaphragm relaxes, moving carbon dioxide up and outward through the chest cavity.

Without optimal contraction and relaxation of the diaphragm, your body compensates to get air in with other muscles, causing imbalances that often lead to pain. What are your breathing habits? Practice awareness. Then get curious, noting how breathing feels and changes when you practice the techniques provided next.

One way to breathe more effectively is to practice an exercise called balloon breathing. This promotes optimal posture and fine-tunes neuromuscular control of 1) the transverse abdominis, 2) the diaphragm, 3) the pelvic floor, and 4) multifidus muscles.

As shown in this illustration, when all these muscles work as a team, they enable optimal activity within your body. They are strong and protect us in activities of daily living.

I've adopted the following exercise from the Postural Restoration Institute™ to provide practical integration of this exercise into your day-to-day living. As you move forward with the 10-Minute Body Maintenance System (chapter 7), this breathing technique will be a cornerstone to your success.

Balloon Breathing Excercise

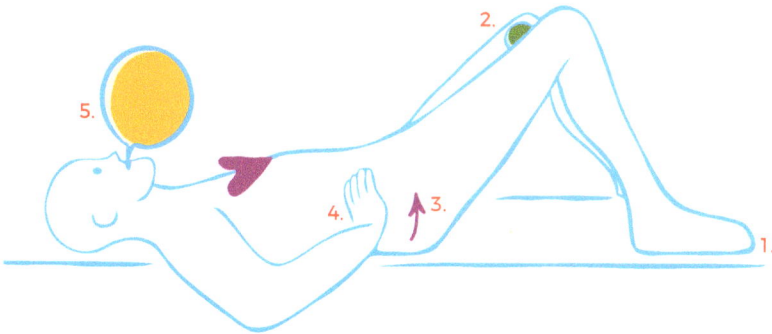

1. Body: lie on your back with your knees bent and feet flat on the floor.
2. Legs: squeeze a 4–6-inch ball or rolled towel between your knees to engage your inner thigh muscles.
3. Back: gently tilt your tailbone toward your belly without lifting your hips off the floor, performing a *posterior pelvic tilt*. Maintain this posterior pelvic tilt for the duration of this exercise.
4. Hands: rest your hands on your lower abdomen.
5. Core: inhale fully through your nose, expanding your belly, and exhale fully through your mouth, blowing air into the balloon (use your imagination if you'd like). Do not release the air from the balloon but rather hold the air in the balloon and breath in through your nose for remaining breaths.
6. Full body: relax all muscles and repeat the inhale-exhale into balloon cycle three to five times, or until the balloon is full.
7. Be curious: as you practice this breathing exercise, see if you can feel your core muscles engage under your hands.

People are often surprised to experience the power of breathing. It helps grow awareness of what's going on in the mind and the body. But mindful breathing also provides the added benefit of calming the heart, mind, and body as a whole, highly integrated system.

By applying or practicing the mindful breathing techniques from this chapter, you promote natural mobility of the body to relieve pain and balance your body.

You can do more formal **mindfulness** practices, too. Although they are beyond the scope of this guidebook, consider exploring options like practicing yoga and other types of bodywork (e.g., massage), or using online resources or apps, like my personal favorite, Headspace®.

The voice of Headspace, Andy Puddicombe, states that "we can't change every little thing that happens to us in life, but we can change the way that we experience it. That's the potential of meditation, of mindfulness. You don't have to burn incense, and you definitely don't have to sit on the floor. All you need to do is to take 10 minutes out a day to step back, to familiarize yourself with the present moment so that you get to experience a greater sense of focus, calm, and clarity in your life."[19]

Mindful breathing can help guide you in developing a greater state of awareness in many aspects of life. But for the purposes of the changes you're making here, it's fundamental to your pain-free living practice and journey. Along the way, your breath can enable greater patience for where you're at, what you notice, and what you feel. By applying or practicing the mindful breathing techniques from this chapter, you promote natural mobility of the body to relieve pain and balance your body.

As you do the following exercises and stretches, bring your breathing into play, using it to create rhythm and help you maximize the movement you're seeking throughout your whole body.

6

Grow Knowledge, Prepare to Move

"Efficiency is concerned with doing things right; effectiveness is doing the right things."

—PETER DRUCKER

n this chapter, we'll keep our breath work in mind as we incorporate additional Tools & Techniques you need to set yourself up for success. Initially, learning these exercises and stretches will require time, practice, and intentional integration into your daily life.

But as you progress, you'll come to feel empowered. You'll know that you're moving toward your potential and possibility. You'll build head-to-toe ability and skill so you can gain sustainable results. Each exercise helps generate a "*shift*," or a change in awareness of a sensation (relief of pain, release of tension, greater mobility, etc.) that gets you closer to how you want to feel in your body.

Let's start by taking a look at proper alignment techniques and their role in creating this positive change.

TECHNIQUES

In building pain-free motion into your life, the first step is to simply learn to stand with what's called the "*aligned standing*" technique. By implementing this simple technique, you'll improve your standing alignment while adjusting your entire body. You'll also help reduce symptoms of Upper and Lower Crossed Syndromes.

So wherever you are, stand up on your two feet to start practicing these five steps of aligned standing. Remember to breathe in through your nose and out through your mouth during each step.

Aligned Standing Technique

Step 1: Neutral Pelvis

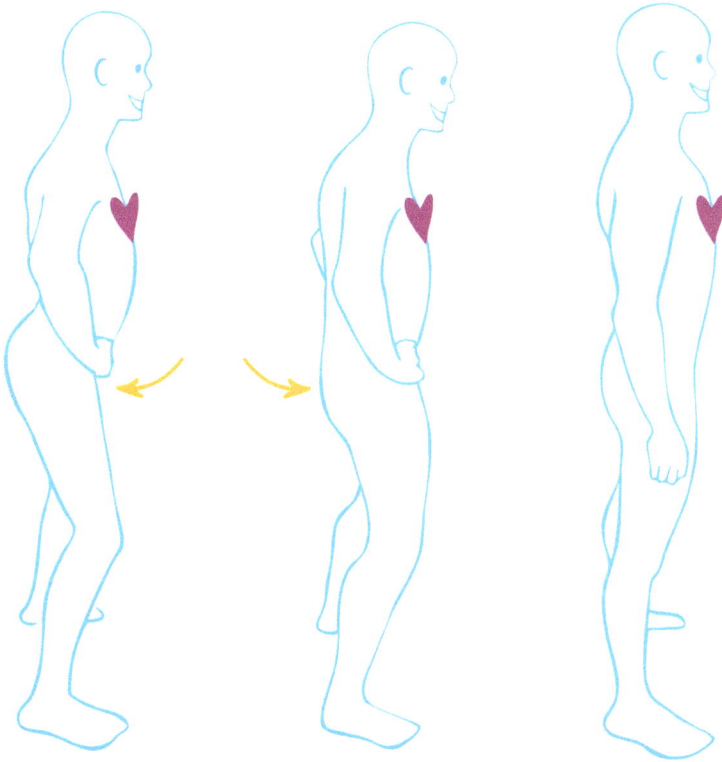

1. Place your feet hip-width apart and point your toes forward.
2. Relax your knees—make sure they're not "locked out."
3. Find your "neutral pelvis," where your pelvis is midway between being tilted all the way forward and backward. To assist you in finding your "neutral pelvis," place your hands on your hips and rock forward and backward six times to loosen up the muscles around your low back, pelvis, and hips. Remember to breathe mindfully.
4. Find a comfortable position in between the two extremes of your pelvis mobility.

Step 2: Spine Stacking

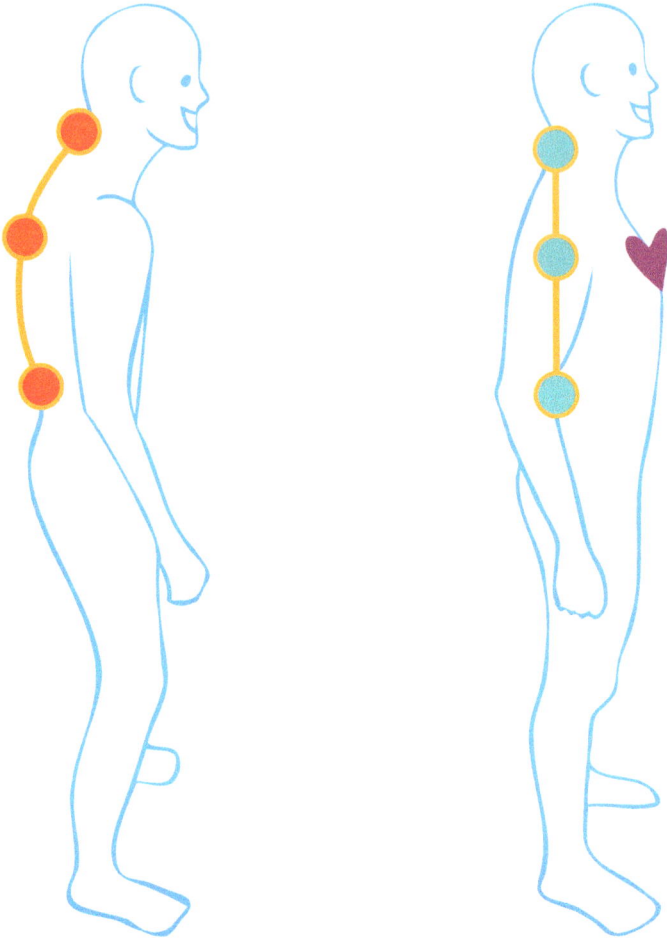

Think about stacking building blocks as you align your spine on top of your neutral pelvis. Picture those blocks as if they are a tall, straight, and sturdy tower.

Step 3: Shoulder Reset

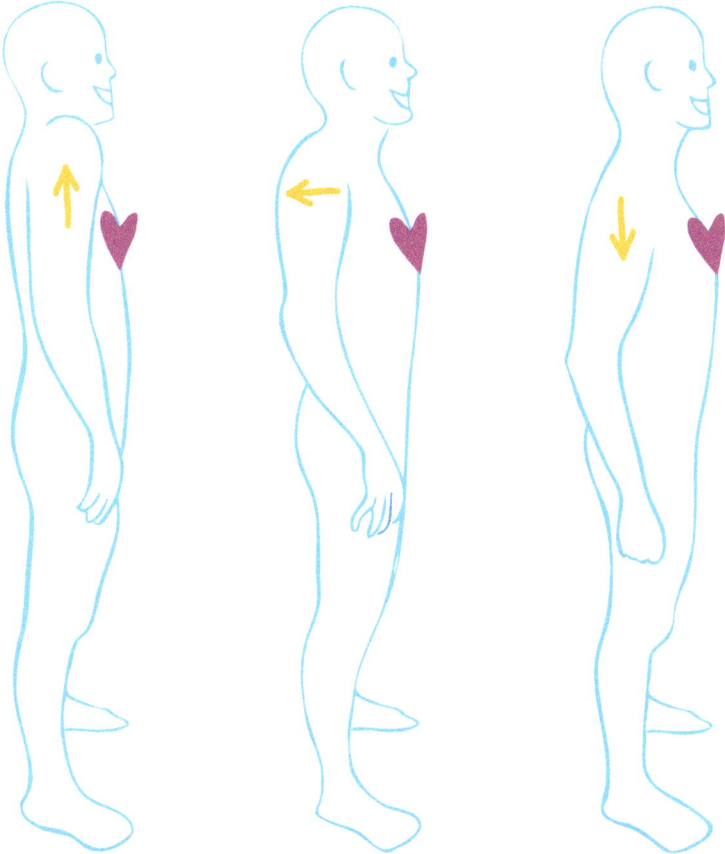

Lift your shoulders toward your ears then roll your shoulder blades back and down.

Step 4: Chin Tuck

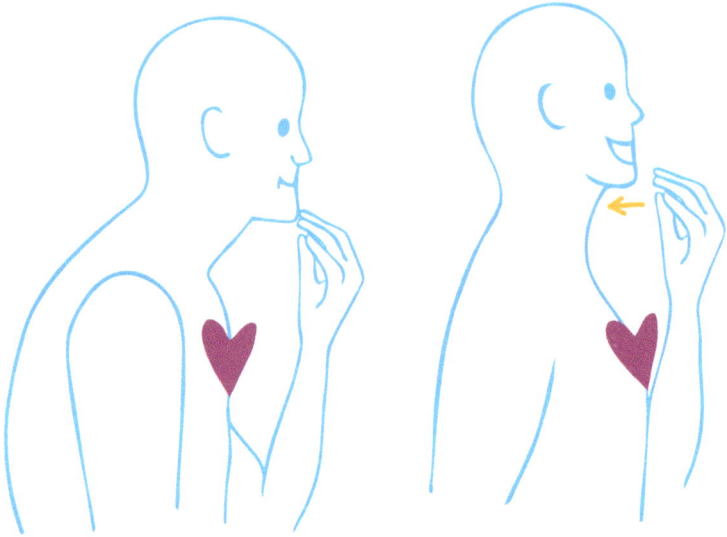

Place your fingertips of one hand on your chin. Keep your eyes looking forward and gently glide your head away from your hand until you feel moderate tension but not pain. This will align your neck and upper back, preventing a hunchbacked position.

Step 5: Final Lift

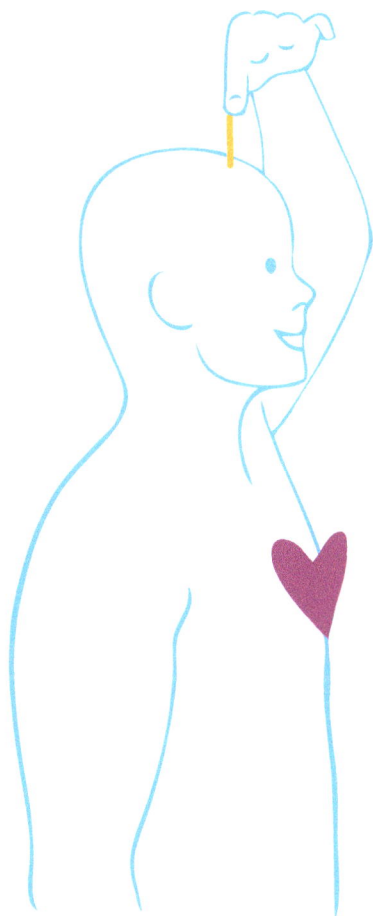

Gently pull the hair on the crown of your head toward the sky until you achieve your final lift.

No matter where you are or why you're standing, check in with your body on a regular basis. Use this aligned standing technique to tweak your real-time, real-world stance so you feel more at ease, energized, and confident in your day.

Aligned Sitting Technique

The steps to aligned standing also apply to **_aligned sitting_**. When you sit, head-to-hip alignment and muscle engagement is still important even though the lower half of your body is essentially "turned off." Go ahead and practice it now, and remember to sit with a neutral pelvis.

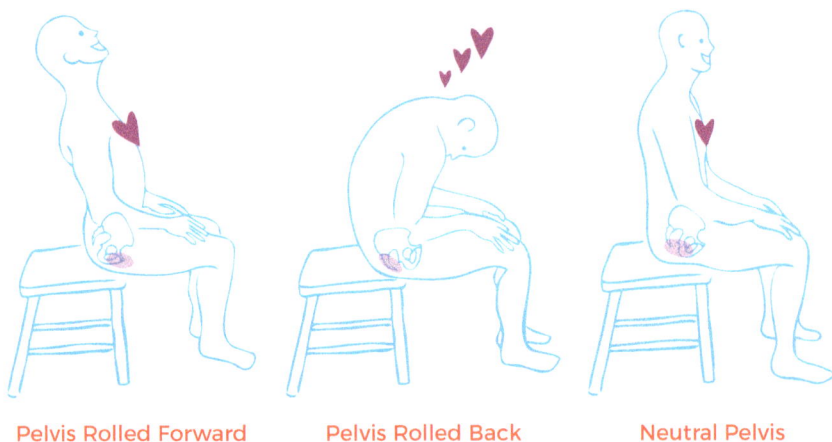

Pelvis Rolled Forward   Pelvis Rolled Back   Neutral Pelvis

1. Sit on the edge of a chair and place your feet flat on the floor.
2. Place your knees at a 90-degree angle or slightly below your hips.
3. Rest your hands on your thighs and roll your hips forward and backward.
4. Find your "neutral pelvis," where your pelvis is midway between being rotated all the way forward and backward. Incorporate your breath to support you.

Now that you know how to sit and stand properly, let's turn to some important tools that build on these alignment concepts while you work.

TOOLS

Active Workstation Design

An **active workstation** is the workspace you design to optimize your body's performance, not break it down. These workstations are commonly called "standing desks," "standing workstations," or "sit-stand workstations." For the purposes of this guidebook, I'm calling them "active workstations" because the goal is to design an active and pain-free lifestyle, not simply to stand more. This solution offers us a way to get up out of our chairs without abandoning our regular lives.

Something as straightforward as standing up or changing positions every 30 minutes while you work can help alleviate both the disease and the dis-ease.

You've probably noticed that when you sit at your desk all day, you feel sluggish, hunched over, and compressed through your spine. Your neck and shoulders feel strained, your mid and low back feel stiff, and your hips are tight. You find yourself shifting in your seat, looking for a comfortable position, and, no matter what you do, you feel bound up, stuck at your desk. It doesn't feel like a disease, but it does feel like *dis*-ease. And yet something as straightforward as standing up or changing positions every 30 minutes while you work can help alleviate both the disease and the dis-ease. Doing a few key stretches and implementing a daily body maintenance system can have an even bigger impact!

Should you really bother with an active workstation or some type of a sit-stand adjustable desk at all? Can you just take more trips to the water cooler or stand more while on the phone to rid yourself of this Sitting Disease? Sure, but as an ambitious, proactive hard worker, you know that the small tweaks and micro-adjustments to your workday can make significant gains over the course of your life.

Any movement helps, but researchers at the Mayo Clinic found that when the study's participants used a sit-stand workstation, they reduced sedentary time, burned more calories, and consumed fewer calories—all of which led to greater health and productivity.[20]

The active workstation provides direct benefits. It improves our activity levels. It enhances our mental, physical, and emotional health. The active workstation supports better digestion and overall body function. In sum, it supports the body's fundamental needs because, after all, we're designed to move.

Whether you're seated, standing, or even leaning, how you align yourself as you move through your day matters. Research shows that aligned sitting, standing, and leaning are vital habits that contribute to a healthy, active lifestyle. As referenced by Lumo Bodytech Inc., innovators of the leading technology-based posture coach, it's the *regular movement* that counts: "Our more nuanced answer about the ideal posture is that 'your next posture is your best posture.'"

In other words, the healthiest thing you can do for your posture is to move as much as possible and avoid maintaining any static posture for an extended period of time. Many of us have jobs that require us to spend time working at desks, so knowing how to sit and stand for good posture is certainly important to our health and well-being. After all, "the human body was built to move, not spend 8 hours at a computer."[21]

The active workstation provides direct benefits. It improves our activity levels. It enhances our mental, physical, and emotional health. The active workstation supports better digestion and overall body function.

Evidence-based science from Ohio State University's Spine Research Institute study suggests the upright leaning workstation is a valid alternative to sitting and standing workstations.[22] Upright leaning offers a dynamic sitting option that promotes a balanced amount of movement, reduces spinal loads, lowers muscle forces, and can be an essential part of a healthy ergonomic workstation design.

Active Workstation Design

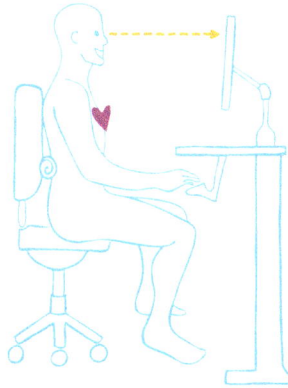

Sit-Stand Desk

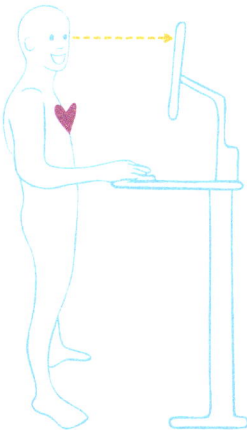

Standing Desk

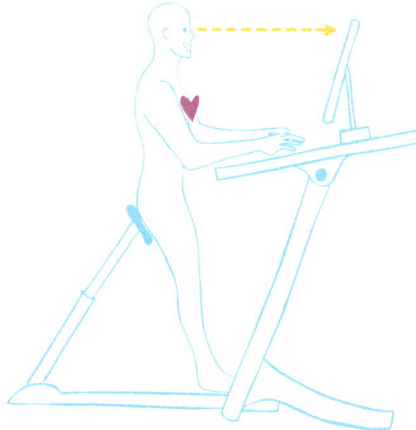

Leaning Desk

In addition to the physical positions, there are a number of "tricks" you can use to easily create an environment that supports your body's alignment. For a DIY trial run, try household items like a couple of textbooks or dictionaries to raise your computer and keyboard while keeping your body upright, engaged, and aligned.

Here is a basic DIY active workstation setup:

DIY Active Workstation Design Checklist

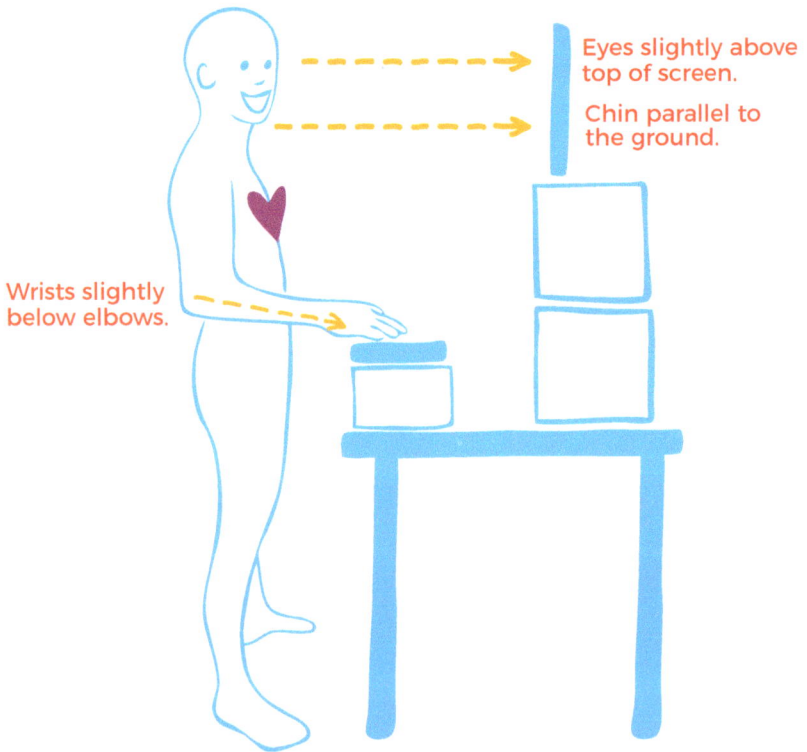

Eyes slightly above top of screen.

Chin parallel to the ground.

Wrists slightly below elbows.

- ✔ Adjustable laptop or monitor riser so top of monitor is slightly below eye level and at arm's length away
- ✔ Wireless keyboard
- ✔ Wireless mouse
- ✔ Wrist support for keyboard and mouse to maintain neutral wrists
- ✔ Anti-fatigue mat
- ✔ Active seat or exercise ball
- ✔ Foot rest and supportive footwear
- ✔ Headset for phone use

Whether you do it yourself or make an investment in an active workstation, the goal is always the same: *fit your workstation to your body, not your body to your workstation.* I have recommended resources on my website, **www.motiontherapy.net**, so you can explore your options and make the best choice for you.

After you've created your active workstation, keep in mind that to support active alignment and recovery for your body, it's important to listen to your body and practice greater awareness. Pay attention to what your body needs regarding your workstation setup as well as your sitting versus standing goals. Then make the changes. In terms of your ultimate standing goal, I recommend working up to standing three additional hours per day, five days a week.

Take time to assess what is working and what's not, practicing curiosity and listening to your body while making steady gains toward your goals. There are no rules—it's all about *your* comfort, preferences, and ability.

TOOLS

Body Maintenance Tools

Regular body maintenance is critical to sustaining the gains you've made in proper alignment and active workstation design. To perform your own body maintenance, your muscles will need a release of knots or sore and painful areas of muscle fibers often referred to as *trigger points*. There are some "body maintenance tools" that can help. You will be incorporating some of these tools into the 10-Minute Body Maintenance System.

I regularly recommend five tools: a Thera Cane, The Stick, a Stretch Out Strap, a foam roller, and a spiky ball. Most people choose one tool that works best for them. Like a pair of shoes, you've got to "try on" the tool you are considering. There is no "one size fits all." If you want to learn more about how to use each tool, you can simply Google the product's manual online. For a more in-depth, customized prescription, I recommend seeing a licensed health-care professional, such as your physical therapist.

The **spiky ball** is a portable self-massage tool that relieves tension in the low back and hips. It fits great in a suitcase, backpack, or purse. All you need is a wall, where you can rub out strains and pains in muscles.

The **Thera Cane** provides relief in the upper back and shoulders, while **The Stick** massages out pain in the legs and low back. Like the spiky ball, the Thera Cane and The Stick are also great tools for people on the go. They can ride along in your car or fit easily in your sports or travel bag.

A **Stretch Out Strap** works on the lower body, including the spine, low back, and toes, while a **foam roller** targets the mid back and the spine, too. They can also help with **nerve gliding**, or muscle stretches that help **soft tissue** move properly and therefore prevent related pain.

Body Maintenance Tools

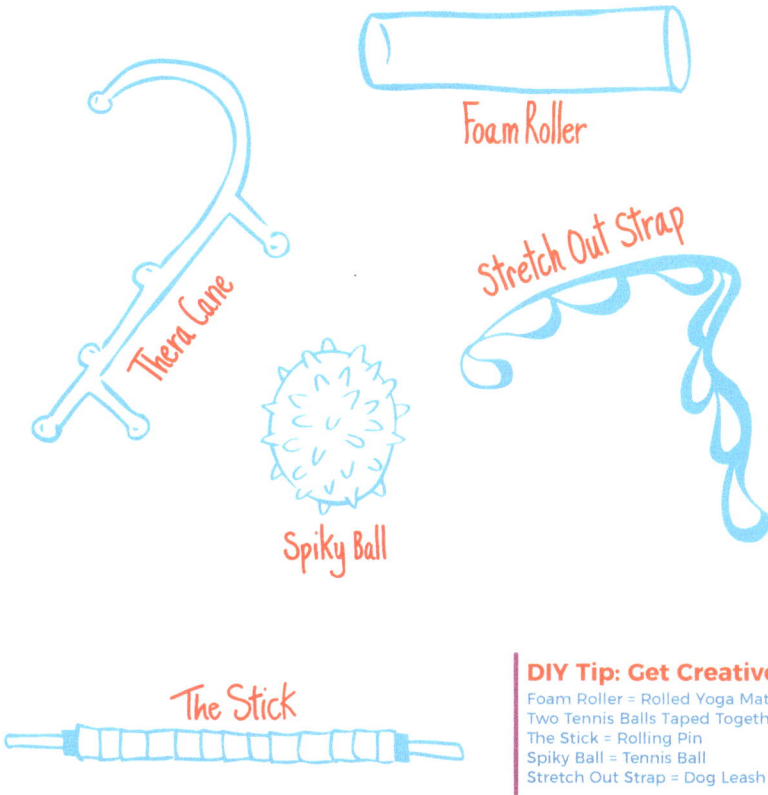

Foam Roller

Thera Cane

Stretch Out Strap

Spiky Ball

The Stick

DIY Tip: Get Creative!
Foam Roller = Rolled Yoga Mat or
Two Tennis Balls Taped Together
The Stick = Rolling Pin
Spiky Ball = Tennis Ball
Stretch Out Strap = Dog Leash

If you prefer a DIY body maintenance tool, I recommend the following:

Foam roller = rolled yoga mat or two tennis balls taped together

The Stick = rolling pin

Spiky ball = tennis ball

Stretch Out Strap = dog leash

Trigger Points + Self-Massage Tools

Spiky Ball
Low Back & Hips

Thera Cane
Upper Back & Shoulders

The Stick
Legs & Low Back

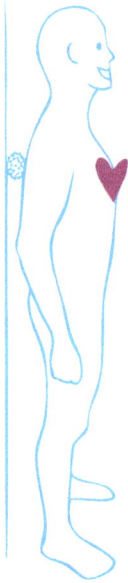
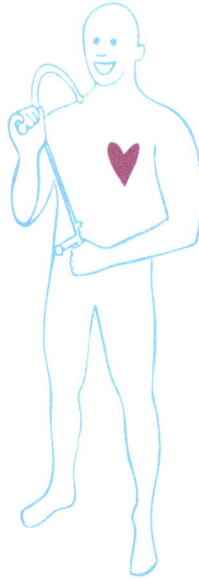
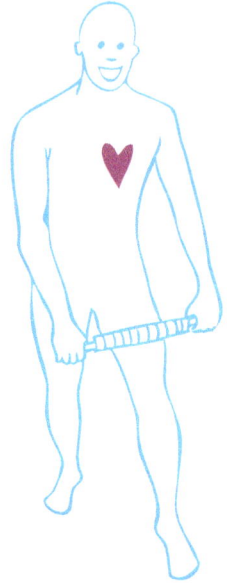

Use these body maintenance tools to self-manage your symptoms. When your body starts screaming for attention, take action and use whichever tool provides your body the most relief for you.

The additional benefit of these tools is that they serve as a visual reminder to do your body maintenance. Practicing with them every day will support you in creating your new active lifestyle habits. When an old, familiar, unwanted sensation comes up, these tools will be there, reminding you to take action.

Here are a few maintenance exercises to try with your Stretch Out Strap and foam roller. These will help you free up trapped lower body nerves, tight muscles, and stiff joints.

Stretch Out Strap: Lower Body Nerve Glide

The subtle motion of this exercise gets to the source of the sensations you're feeling, gently elongating tight muscles, gliding nerves, and realigning spinal segments.

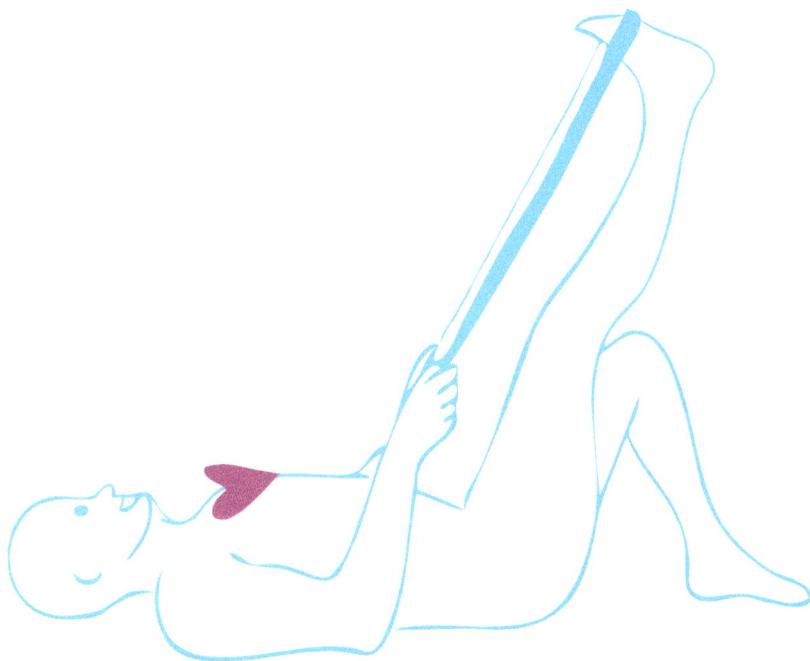

1. Body: lie on your back with knees bent and feet on the ground.
2. Leg: place strap loop around the ball of your foot and gently straighten your knee. Be sure to keep your knee and ankle locked through this exercise.
3. Foot: gently pull your foot toward the sky until you feel a good amount of tension, but not pain, along the hip, knee, and foot. Next, release the foot in the strap just enough to release the stretch. Repeat 10 times and then switch to the other side.
4. Be curious: breathe and explore your range of motion by gently pulling the strap across or away from your midline. What do you feel and where?

Foam Roller: Mid Back Mobility

Using the foam roller, focus on building greater flexibility and mobility around the mid back region. This tool massages back muscles and mobilizes segments of the spine. My clients often describe the feeling of traction or elongation of the spine providing greater mobility after long bouts of sitting.

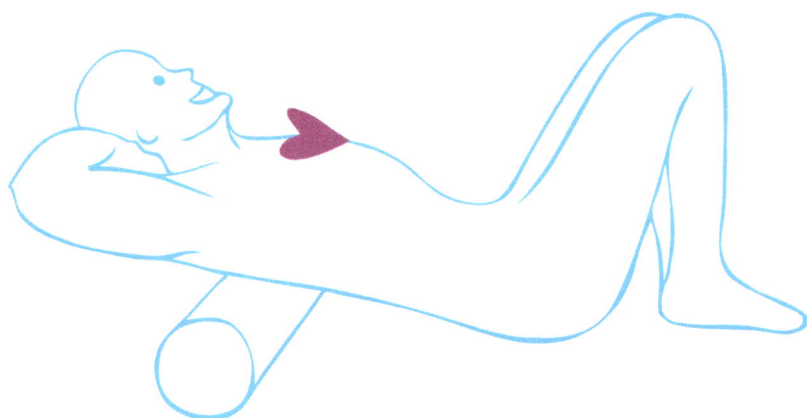

1. Body: lie on your back and extend your mid spine over the foam roller.
2. Hips + Knees: bend your hips and knees, keeping your hips and feet on the ground.
3. Neck: clasp your hands behind your neck to support your head.
4. Be curious: gently extend your spine over the foam roller as you take six breaths. Each breath ought to help you relax tight muscles and extend your mid back farther over the foam roller. What do you feel and where?

Foam Roller: Lower Body Mobility

Now roll out the back of your hips, inner and outer thighs, and inner and outer lower leg, smoothing out tight muscles and relieving areas of tension throughout the lower body.

Enjoy the slight twist of your upper body as you turn toward the ground. This rotation of your body will enhance arm and core strength as you move through this foam roller exercise.

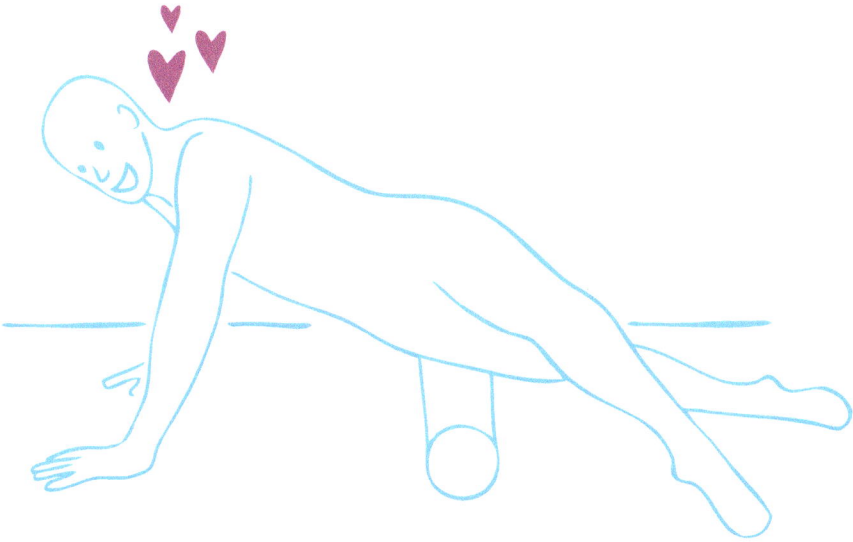

1. Arms: prop yourself on the foam roller near the region of your symptoms.
2. Body: use your body weight to deliver sustainable pressure to your body; this will release trigger points, knots, and tension in muscles.
3. Be curious: roll your body weight on and off the region of your symptoms. Breathe and notice; what do you feel and where?

Now that you have the foundational Tools & Techniques you need to resolve body pain caused by excessive sitting, it's time to look at how you'll incorporate these into the 10-Minute Body Maintenance System.

7

Power Up Your Practice

"Don't wish it were easier,
wish you were better."

—JIM ROHN

B y now, you've got a solid understanding of the techniques and tools that will support you in getting out of your chair and not just sitting there. You are now ready for the 10-Minute Body Maintenance System.

Why a "system"? Creating and implementing a system is the vital strategy for sustaining your pain-free, active lifestyle. This system consists of 10 specific, science-backed techniques that target imbalances from long hours of sitting. While these exercises have a number of benefits, we're using them to address the most common imbalances resulting in Upper and Lower Crossed Syndromes (see the beginning of Part II). Over the last decade of working one-on-one with people, I've found that the following stretching techniques are simple, practical, and many times provide immediate relief from the symptoms that result from these two syndromes.

This system is so powerful because it takes a small amount of time and can be done almost anywhere. You don't need to go the gym, purchase weights, or sign up for boot camp. Throughout your day, you simply need to move your own body, perform daily maintenance, and maintain proper alignment.

The *convenience* of this system is what will empower you to remain *consistent* in your *commitment* to this new active-lifestyle habit.

The system is also customizable based on how *you feel*. You don't have to do every exercise every day, nor do you have to use all the tools. Once you've learned the system, you're free to spend 10 minutes a day with the technique and tool that provides the relief you need.

STRATEGY

The 10-Minute Body Maintenance System

The following 10 body maintenance exercises are arranged to target imbalances from head to toe. So, I recommend beginning with the first technique on day one and practicing it for 10 minutes. Then, practice a new technique for 10 minutes each day. After 10 days, you'll have learned and practiced each of the 10 stretching techniques. You will have effectively taken your body through its initial run of the head-to-toe Body Maintenance System.

Along with the daily exercise, choose a body maintenance tool to incorporate into your 10 minutes. As mentioned in the last chapter, I usually encourage my clients to test out each of the five tools to know which one best targets their pain. To use the tools, simply choose from the three stretches I mentioned in chapter 6 or pick from the tool's guide, depending on your specific pain.

As you practice each exercise and stretch with each tool, pay attention to how your body responds and how you feel. After you've moved through all 10 techniques, you should have a good idea of which techniques and tools address your pain. Going forward, you can choose one technique and one tool depending on what your body is telling you—whether that's shoulder pain, neck strain, low back tension, or another form of pain. Then, practice the specific stretching technique (for the region of your pain) and use your body maintenance tool of choice for just 10 minutes every day. Some of my clients continue working through the entire system to regularly target all their imbalances. And since the body continually changes, some customize the system over time by switching out the technique and tool they use daily.

After 10 days, you'll have learned and practiced each of the 10 stretching techniques. You will have effectively taken your body through its initial run of the head-to-toe Body Maintenance System.

Understandably so, the system will not be completed in 10 minutes on the first day. Once you've learned the skills and increased your ability to integrate the system into your day, you will find that 10 minutes is a doable and sustainable amount of time to keep performing the system daily. Your skills, ability, and consistency in taking daily action to apply the system, along with the body maintenance tools, set the foundation for sustaining your pain-free posture.

The 10-Minute Body Maintenance System becomes a new habit:

- that you do at least once a day
- that takes you only 10 minutes
- that requires little effort once the knowledge is gained

As you move through each technique, practice mindful breathing. Pay attention to exactly how your body feels when you breathe in and out.

Let's get started!

Neck Stretch

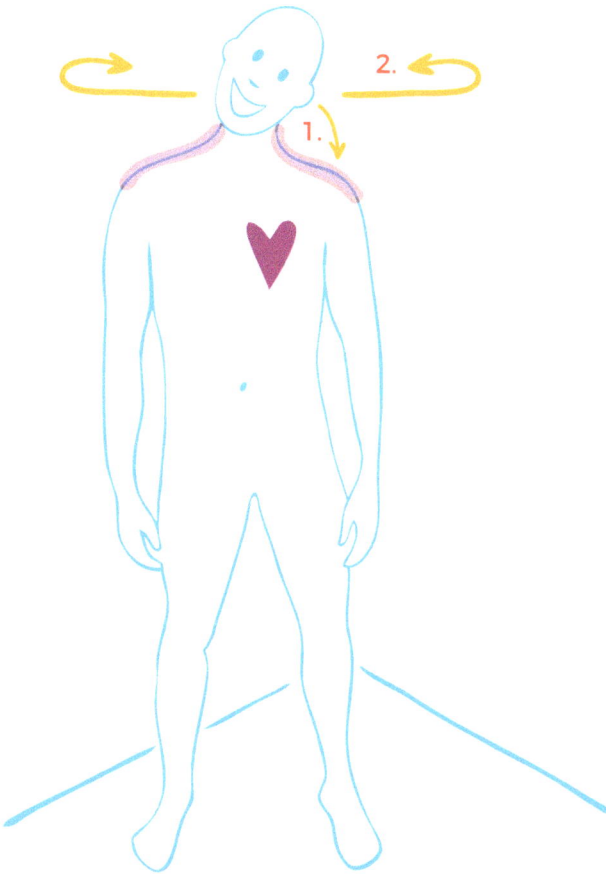

Because you're moving your neck in ways you may not be used to, this stretch won't likely be felt just in your neck. If you're like many people, you may experience stretching or releasing sensations from the neck to the top of the shoulders, around the base of your neck, and down your upper back. Don't worry; this is normal.

1. Neck: with your eyes looking forward, tilt your right ear toward the right shoulder and hold for six breaths. Switch and repeat on the other side.

2. Neck: with your eyes looking forward, turn your head to the right and hold for six breaths. Switch and repeat on the other side.
3. Neck: gaze down to your armpit and hold for six breaths. Switch and repeat on the other side.
4. Be curious: Breathe and notice; what do you feel and where?

Upper Body Nerve Glide

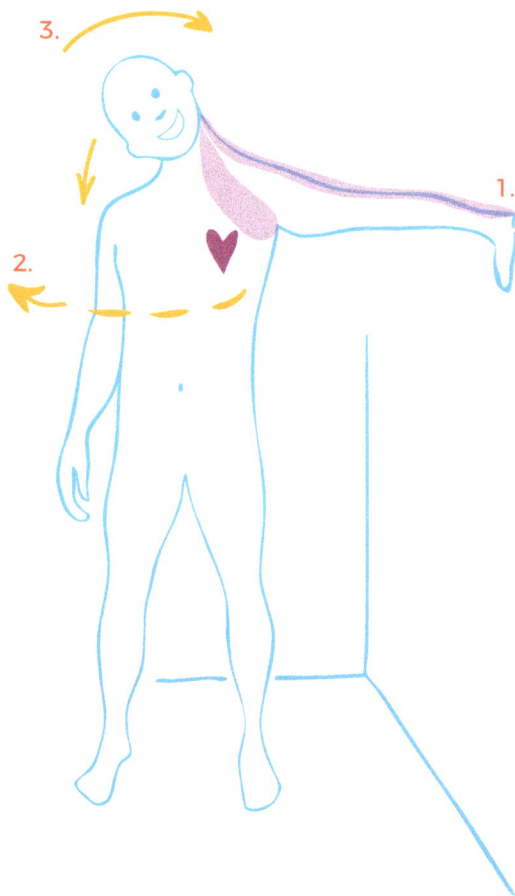

Bring your neck, arm, wrist, hand, and even fingertips alive with this simple exercise. Avoid sharp pain at the edge of your comfort zone, but embrace the intensity of this stretch as it may be felt from your neck all the way down your arm, forearm, and into your fingers. It is normal to feel intense stretching as you glide the nerve through the soft tissue of your entire arm.

1. Arm: gently press the palm of your right hand on the wall with your fingers reaching down toward the ground at a level between your belly button and shoulder. Gently extend your elbow.
2. Body: maintain the arm position and rotate your body slightly away from the wall.
3. Neck: tilt your ear toward the left shoulder and return the head to center 10 times. DO NOT HOLD the stretch but rather gently move between the tilted position to neutral 10 times. Switch to the other side (left hand on wall) and repeat the same steps.
4. Be curious: breathe and notice; what do you feel and where?

Chest Opener Stretch

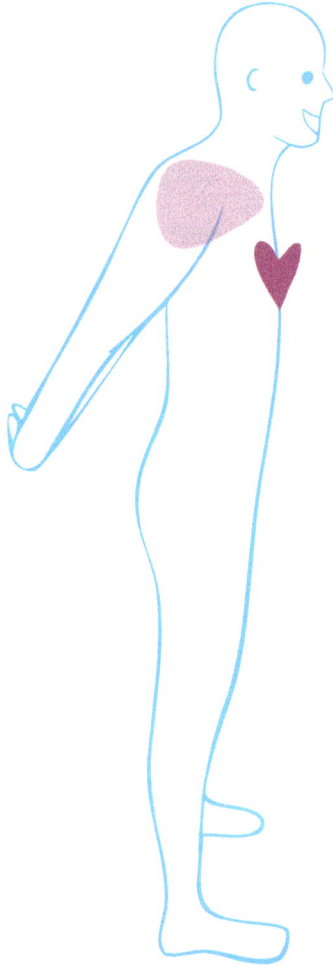

With this chest opener, expect a domino effect of sensations to run from your neck to your mid to upper arm and into your forearm and hand.

1. Hands: clasp your hands together behind your back.
2. Arms: lift your clasped hands away from your low back until you feel a good amount of tension but not pain; hold for six breaths.
3. Be curious: breathe and notice; what do you feel and where?

Shoulder Reset Stretch

This stretch turns on a collection of muscles that aren't worked often in people suffering from prolonged sitting or Upper Crossed

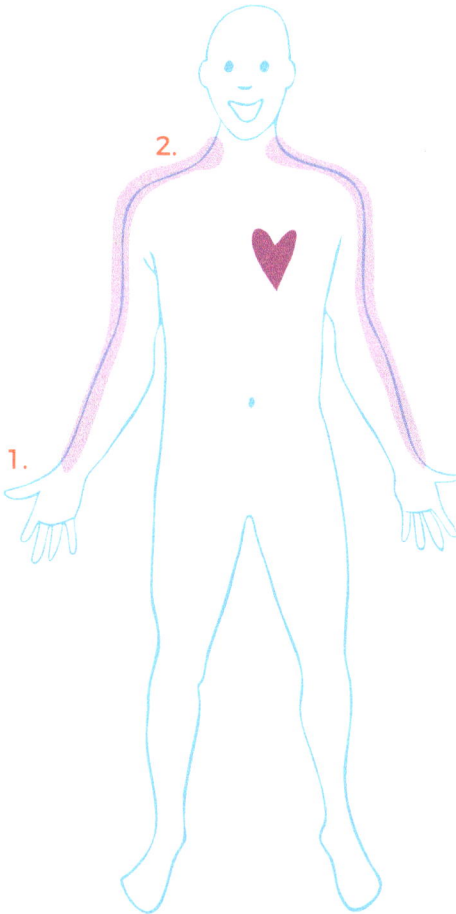

Syndrome. Allowing your chest to fully expand also engages the muscles in your upper back.

Sometimes, in holding this stretch, fatigue can set into your back muscles. This isn't just normal—it's a good thing. Embrace it, breathe into it.

1. Body: stand with your palms facing forward, slightly away from your body, with your hands reaching toward the ground and your chin tucked.
2. Shoulder blades: gently squeeze your shoulders back and downward. Maintain your chin tuck and hold for six breaths.
3. Be curious: breathe and notice; what do you feel and where?

Shoulders + Mid Back Stretch

You will likely find this exercise to be the most challenging. Move into it slowly, mindfully, and deliberately. The movements in this

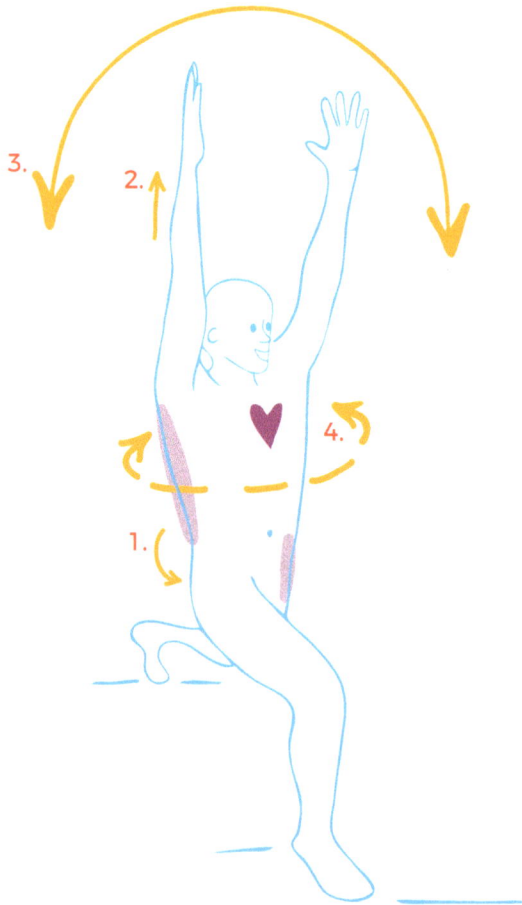

exercise activate the entire body head to toe rather than in its separate parts.

1. Body: assume lunge position, trunk upright, core engaged, tailbone tucked under.
2. Hands: reach your hands overhead toward the sky and hold for six breaths. Keep your shoulders relaxed.
3. Hands: with your hands still above you, bend to the left side and right side as if your upper body is between two planes of glass. Again, six breaths on each side.
4. Hands: reach in front of you at chest level and rotate until you feel a good amount of tension, but not pain, in both directions. Hold for six breaths on each side.
5. Legs: Switch legs now, repeating this exercise on the other side.
6. Be curious: breathe and notice; what do you feel and where?

Seated Spine Stretch

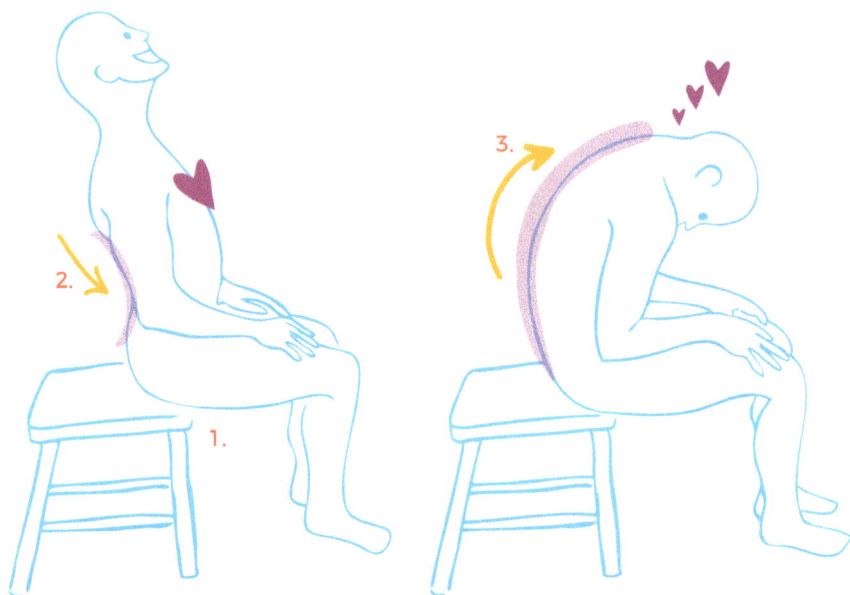

If you hear a little "snap, crackle, and pop" during this stretch, don't be alarmed! It's your spine and muscles releasing and resetting as they move through a broader range of motion. Reset your spine regularly, doing this little exercise while you're seated at your desk, on a plane, in front of your TV, etc.

1. Body: sit on the edge of your chair with your hands on your thighs.
2. Hips: inhale, tilting your pelvis forward, gently arching your low back, reaching your chest to the sky.
3. Hips: exhale, tilting your pelvis backward, gently rounding your low back and letting your head relax toward your chest.
4. Be curious: follow the movement of your breath as you repeat the forward and backward movement of your pelvis six times. What do you feel and where?

Piriformis Stretch

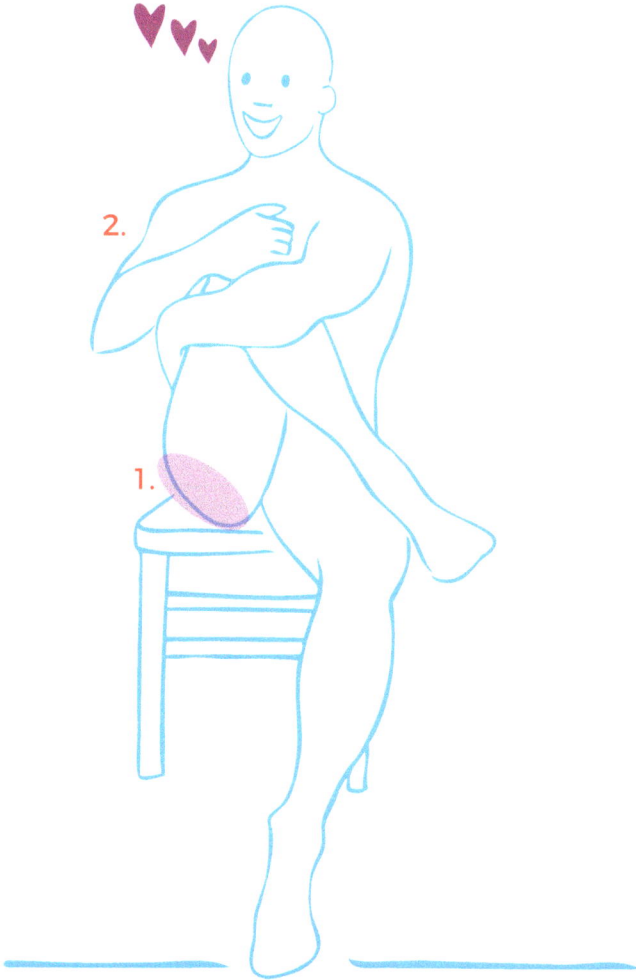

Make your hips come alive with this oh-so-good, deep posterior hip stretch. By lengthening bound-up hip muscles, this exercise releases persistent pulling in the low back and hip after prolonged sitting.

1. Body: sit on the edge of your chair and place one ankle on your opposite thigh or shin. Stay tall in your trunk.
2. Hips: maintain "neutral pelvis" and hug your knee toward the opposite shoulder. Hold for six breaths. Switch to the other side and repeat with your other knee. NOTE: If you feel pinching in the hip that you are hugging, release your hug to avoid pinching the soft tissue in your hip.
3. Be curious: gently twist your spine toward the knee you are hugging. Breathe and notice; what do you feel and where?

Hamstring + Low Back Stretch

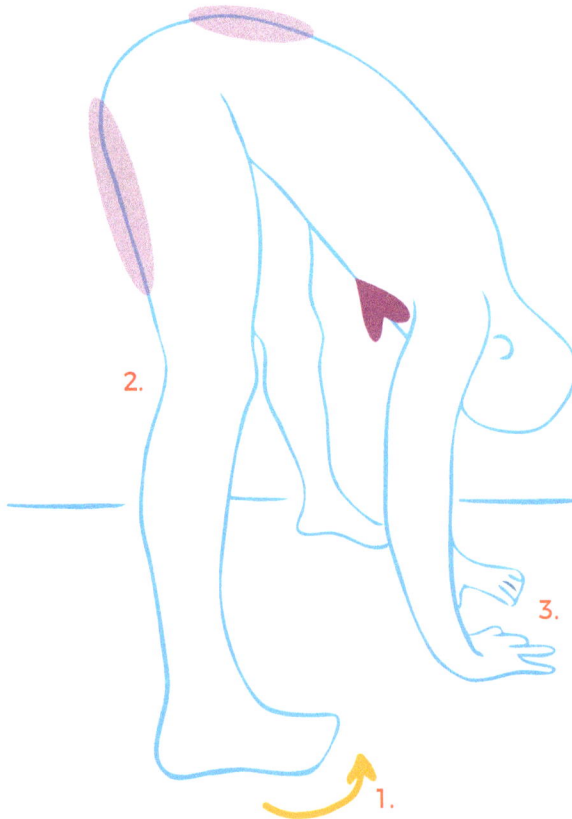

This stretch uses self-created traction to bring a cascade of relief from the outer hips down through your legs and into your toes. Meanwhile, the back, neck, and spine are unloaded by using your own body weight. This stretching technique is natural, gentle traction at its best!

1. Feet: spread your feet a little wider than hip-width apart. Turn your toes inward.
2. Body: from an upright stance position, walk your hands down your body, creating a forward fold from your hips. If your hands do not reach the floor, support your trunk with your hands on your shins.
3. Legs: gently straighten both your knees and hold for six breaths.
4. Be curious: reach your hands to the outside of both of your feet. Breathe and notice; what do you feel and where?

Hip + Quad Stretch

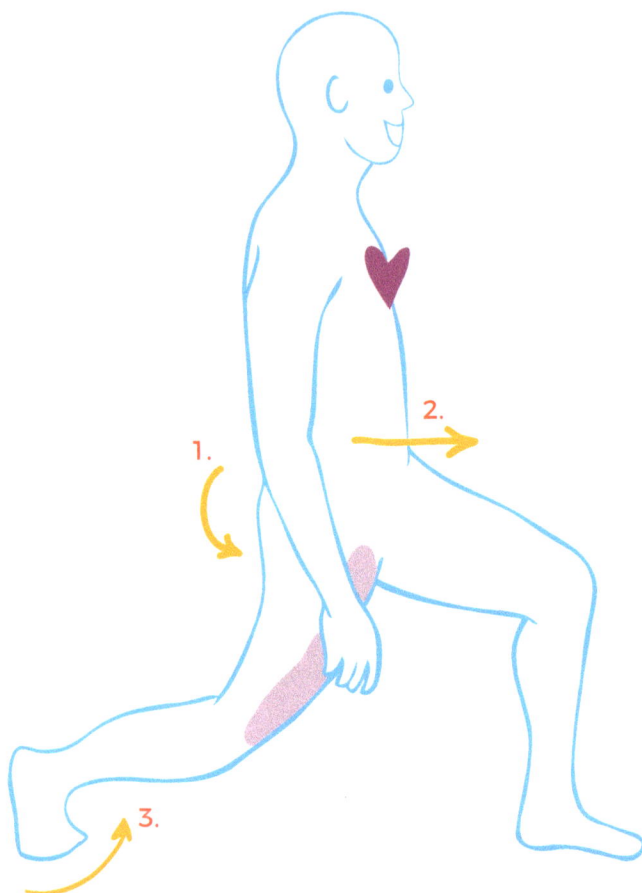

Be sure to maintain your upper body alignment as you step into this challenging stretch, which targets the front of the hip, inner thigh, lower leg, and low back muscles. With just a little rotation of the foot inward, you'll elongate the tight muscles at the front of your hip.

1. Body: assume lunge position, core engaged, trunk upright, tailbone tucked under.
2. Hips: square your hips so they are both facing forward.
3. Back foot: turn your toes inward and hold for six breaths. Switch to the other side and repeat.

4. Be curious: tilt your pelvis forward and backward to find your "neutral pelvis." Breathe and notice; what do you feel and where?

Calf + Lower Leg Stretch

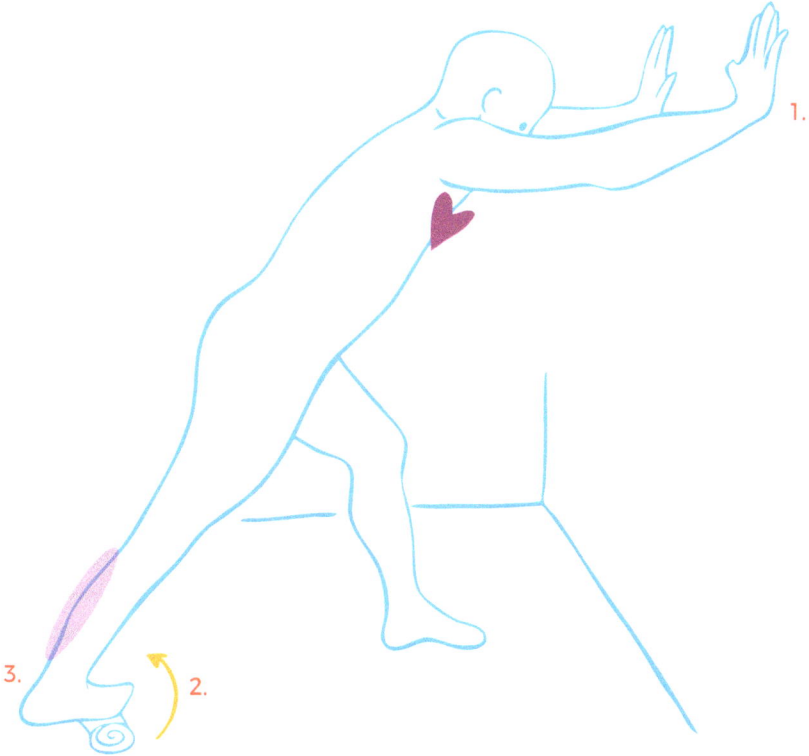

Not everyone thinks to stretch out the calf and lower leg to relieve spine and body strain. Allow this exercise to reengage those oft-ignored muscles. You'll wake up a number of tight muscles, lengthening them from right behind and around the knee, down into your calf, and around your foot.

1. Body: facing a wall, step into a lunge position, with your hands touching the wall.
2. Back leg: put the ball of your foot on an approximately

three-inch towel roll with your toes turned inward. A hand towel works great.
3. Back leg: push your heel into the ground and hold for six breaths. Switch to the other side and repeat.
4. Be curious: breathe as you turn your toes slightly more inward. What do you feel and where?

You did it! By learning and applying these 10 stretching techniques, you have a daily system for head-to-toe body maintenance. With each of these stretching techniques, remember that practice makes progress. It's not about permanence or perfection. With just 10 minutes a day of taking action and practicing these stretching techniques, you can create a new habit and make this system part of your active, pain-free lifestyle.

At minimum, you are now aware that body maintenance is critical to achieving the sensations, body state, and feelings you desire (Part I). And you now have a practical, specific prescription—the 10-Minute Body Maintenance System—to live pain-free, energized, and confident. Now I challenge you to make this system a routine part of your workday so that you can truly achieve and live your desired results and outcomes!

PART III

Results & Outcomes

Now you know the tools, techniques, and strategies to live and sustain your pain-free life. Yet do you find you're struggling to make it all part of your day-to-day life? Does it all feel difficult because of limited time, money, or other barriers that are discouraging you from achieving your goals? What exactly is getting in your way?

Replace the excuse making with a good habit, one that moves you from pain to possibility.

I'm willing to guess that some of you are struggling with daily, consistent application of your new knowledge and skills. When other people tell me about their resistance, I hear statements like:

I don't have time.
I'm too busy.
It's impossible for me to do it alone.
I don't have the energy.
I am afraid I will make my pain worse.
I don't have the support I need.

I don't have enough money.
I don't know where to start.

Do any of these common statements sound familiar to you? At times, we all try to justify why we cannot make a change.

From my own experience, I have always found the resources necessary to support my desires. Don't get me wrong. I catch myself making plenty of excuses. I have even created deliberate routines with clear cues to remind myself of my vision and how I want to live my pain-free life. And sometimes I still struggle, coming up with some excuse or another.

However, here's the reality: Making excuses is a bad habit. So I course-correct, focusing on my goals that align with my lifelong vision. And then it's about taking little steps and giving my best effort.

And so, too, can you do this. Replace the excuse making with a good habit, one that moves you from pain to possibility. The key to navigating bumps in the road and working around roadblocks is all about reconnecting to your vision.

8

Act with Accountability to Sustain Momentum

"Set a goal, and in small, consistent steps, work to reach it. Get support from your peers when you start flagging. Repeat. You will change."

—SETH GODIN

M any people say that adopting habits to create a healthier lifestyle affects different aspects of their life. When they make decisions that align with their vision, their actions produce a growing sense of purpose and vitality. They become more aware of their intuition. They gain clarity and confidence in their purpose, which drives greater self-initiative. They feel invigorated with newfound knowledge and abilities to manage their pain independently. Ultimately, this is all about transformation—even freedom. Instead of feeling pain, they realize they're focused on possibility. Their pain isn't *pushing* them. Their possibility is *pulling* them.

You can find your freedom by becoming your own guide. Own your ability (and responsibility) to move toward your goals. Yet even with this sense of ownership, having accountability will be essential to your success.

In helping people achieve their goals, I've noticed that having a buddy is the best way for them to remain accountable. So if you are struggling with commitment, you may benefit from the support of an accountability partner or even a group.

Having accountability will be essential to your success.

For example, consider working with a physical therapist, yoga therapist, personal trainer, athletic trainer, or health coach. But if for any reason this option isn't for you, or if you don't want to ask a friend or colleague to help you, don't beat yourself up about it. Consider a membership at a yoga studio, join the local sports club, or sign up for seasonal intramural groups. After all, people are hardwired for connection. With a group, the connection, community, and unity toward a common goal create belief—namely, the belief that you can accomplish your goals. This is the power of groups and shared experiences.

Tracking Your Health Progress

It's also important to track your progress toward your goals. As your guide, I've developed a Healthy Habit Tool that you can start using immediately. Keep this tracking tool handy so you can conveniently monitor your progress. Simply mark a "Y" or "N" in each box if you have completed the 10-Minute Body Maintenance System for the day. You can also use it to track other goals, such as standing for three hours during your workday. Then mark a happy, neutral, or sad smiley face depending on how you felt that day while working toward your goal. (see note in Appendix)

If you prefer tracking your progress in another way, that's perfectly fine. You can journal, use an app on your smartphone (such as Way of Life, Momentum, and My Habits), or invest in a wearable fitness tracker to create accountability. The point is to do something! Take action.

Goal: 10-Minute Body Maintenance

Motion Therapy	Week 1	Week 2	Week 3	Week 4	Week 5	Week 6	Week 7	Week 8	Week 9	Week 10
Monday										
Tuesday										
Wednesday										
Thursday										
Friday										
Saturday										
Sunday										
Done on 5 days? Y or N										
How natural did it feel? ☺ ☺ ☹										

Finally, you can also boost your odds of success through **self-pacing and graded exposure**. These are perhaps best discussed in *Explain Pain*, a neuroscience and pain education book I love to reference when working with clients. In the chapter entitled "Pacing and Graded Exposure," the authors outline five ways to pace yourself effectively.[23] Below, I've summarized the steps and adapted them to the context here:

1. **Choose what you'll do more.** Pick a specific activity that's challenging for you, like standing at your workstation for three hours per day, five days a week, over the next two weeks.

2. **Note your baseline.** How much of the activity you've chosen can you do without a flare-up, such as pain or some other symptom? Whatever you can "definitely" do without pain, symptoms, or feeling desperate, this is your baseline. Use it as your starting point, or what you'll build upon at first.

3. **Plan your progression.** The point is to make incremental improvements toward your goal while being patient with yourself. If you walked 15 minutes today without pain

symptoms, you may try 17 minutes tomorrow, 19 minutes the next day, 21 minutes the day after that, etc. Plan ahead for this progressive, conscientious style of improvement, and it will feel more doable both mentally and physically. You'll be guaranteed to experience little wins along the way. Even just making the effort to create your plan can also provide you with a feeling of personal *wow!*

4. **Accept any flare-ups.** Pain is not the goal, so if you notice you're suddenly flaring up, it's your body's alarm telling you that enough is enough—for now. Pay attention to it. Honor that honest communication. Don't give up on the practice you've adopted, but scale back until you've recovered, then step it up a notch once again. Don't quit your activity—keep trying, and your body will eventually embrace this change.

5. **Make it your lifestyle.** No doubt, you'll have to plan your life a bit more, but the activities you're choosing to do, or the habits you're now adopting, will bring you joy, even if it's just small bursts of joy. Schedule these activities into what you're doing on a more regular basis. Invite friends and family members to join and support you when you can. These folks don't need to be your official accountability partners; ask anyone you like or love to join in on your fun! Over time, you'll come to believe this is simply who you are and what you do.

Whatever you do, make accountability and checking-in a habit that's convenient for you. Otherwise, you'll struggle. When you keep the momentum going over the long haul, you'll be more likely to sustain your active lifestyle habits.

9

Embrace the 3Cs— Commitment, Convenience, and Consistency

"We are what we repeatedly do.
Excellence, then, is not an act but a habit."

—ARISTOTLE

t never fails. When a client experiences a win with immediate relief, makes progress, and generates momentum toward living injury-free and pain-free, they often ask, "What do I need to do next?" Here's what I say:

Sustainable gains are achieved by practicing good habits.

Sustainable gains are achieved by practicing good habits. Like many of my clients, you are creating new habits, and the choices, activities, and behaviors that you repeatedly practice become your lifestyle. There will be bumps in the road, even unforeseen roadblocks. If you want to feel better, however, you will need to dig deep for the willpower and strength to keep practicing the right habits. To do that with success requires relentless focus on what I call the "3Cs."

- You honor this process with **Commitment**
- You make your habits **Convenient**
- You practice them with **Consistency**

Marie Forleo, one of my online marketing mentors, regularly says, "Clarity comes through engagement, not thought."[24] So you have to take action and engage with your *commitments*, find ways to *conveniently* integrate the best practices into your daily living, and *consistently* move toward achieving your goals.

Here's a breakdown of the 3Cs:

COMMITMENT. This is about doing what you've promised yourself you will do. You've already created clarity around your vision and set goals. And, you've also committed to learning the Tools & Techniques that will empower you to achieve greater health, happiness, and performance. But sustaining your commitment requires that you reengage with it regularly. It requires staying inspired on a daily basis. Everybody's approach to this will be unique, but here are some activities I recommend for maintaining a daily commitment to your health and wellness vision:

- **Address what's working and what's not.** Pay close attention to when and how you've been successful relative to your goals. When you've come up short, what's going on? What steps can you take to address any obstacles so you're regularly committed to achieving what you want to feel—that possibility you desire and deserve?

- **Be intentional and deliberate.** Good intentions are meaningless if you don't take purposeful action. Use your SMART goals to take you in the direction of your health and wellness vision. Design your life, be intentional, and take deliberate action in your day-to-day activities.

- **Practice gratitude**. Be grateful for the health and wellness that you have at this moment. Yes, we can improve in some or many areas of our life. At the moment, you are breathing, reading, and reflecting on these strategies, and it is important to practice gratitude for where you are right now.

- **Practice visualization.** Use your mind's eye to imagine your active, healthy, vibrant self. Visualization is a powerful tool allowing you to "see" your pain-free body, know your mindset, and feel your spirit, all free of dis-ease and full of life, energy, and self-confidence.

CONVENIENT. Let's face it—if something isn't convenient to do, then we're less likely to do it, period. So it's essential to develop ways to make your habit realistic or practical to do. Here are some ideas for boosting the convenience factor:

- **Learn to use your excuses.** We often make excuses for why we aren't achieving our goals. Usually those excuses relate to the fact that it's inconvenient to do something, *It's essential to develop ways to make your habit realistic or practical to do.* even though we know it will improve our ability to succeed. If you're making excuses, don't judge or criticize yourself for it. But do note and use them to take corrective action and address the issues. For example, if you are making a lot of excuses in regard to time, then that's your cue that you've got an activity-management issue you need to address if you're going to make progress toward your goal.

- **Check in on your alignment.** No matter where you are or what you're doing, you can easily self-assess your alignment and course-correct if you're off track. You can also take a photo of yourself at your desk or workstation. Using this visual image, quickly determine how you "stack up" in regard to the alignment techniques you've learned. Go back to the section with aligned standing and aligned sitting for a quick check.

- **Assess your active workstation.** Is it working? For example, is your exercise ball collecting dust in a nearby closet? Switch out your chair for the ball instead. If you're finding you're not using your workstation because there are some issues with the height, do the necessary remodeling or grab a stack of books to lift up your monitor to eye level. (See five steps in Chapter 6 for aligned sitting and standing.) The point is to do it all correctly so using these tools becomes easier and more convenient than not using them.
- **Invest in an active workstation.** Wanting to upgrade from a DIY version of your active workstation to something that perhaps has more style, functionality, or flexibility? You're in luck. Go to my website (motiontherapy.net) to access additional resources.
- **"Plant" tools in familiar places.** For example, you can purchase an active seat, put it in your living room, and use it when you watch your favorite shows. Or as we discussed earlier, you can do things like deliberately place your foam roller on the bedroom floor so it becomes incorporated into your nightly routine. If you've got a Thera Cane, you can also put it in your car's middle console so it's easy to grab and use after a long drive. It's easy enough to place a spiky ball in your shower. Using it to give yourself a mini massage will become the "excuse" you need to spend that extra five minutes under the hot water.

CONSISTENCY. In addition to commitment and convenience, being consistent with your mindset and behaviors is a vital key to achieving your goals. In a podcast interview featured in Lewis Howes's *The School of Greatness*, John Maxwell states,

"Consistency will give you a compounding that no other trait will." Like compound interest, its exponential growth leads to significant gains.[25]

Here are a few ways to improve consistency:

- **Use reminders and/or cues.** Starting new practices and changing up a routine can be tough. But if you simply get started, you'll find you're much more motivated to follow through. The trick is to figure out ways to trigger your new, good habits, such as:

    ✔ *Through your active workstation of choice*, for example, the standing desk plus a yoga/exercise ball for your seated desk and a spiky ball on the surface of your workstation. Even something as simple as sticky notes with reminders to move on the half-hour can help.

    ✔ *With active lifestyle technology* by trying your favorite apps. Consider those like UpDesk and Stand Up!, for example. Or you might check out resources like juststand.org and give wearable tools like a fitness tracker, iWatch, or Lumo Lift a try.

    ✔ *By practicing greater body awareness*, to acknowledge and listen to your body. Practice being present with your body's sensations. What are they telling you? To hydrate? Move? Take a break? Do it!

- **Implement an accountability system.** Designing your accountability plan is a great first step. But then you've got to implement it. Take that critical action!

- **Schedule a "progress report,"** ideally every 14 days, to reflect, self-check, and measure your progress toward your SMART goals. You can also plan a weekly, monthly, or quarterly meeting with your mentor, coach, or accountability partner to maintain your momentum toward your goals. Progress reports are a proven method for consistently tracking your success. You can place a reminder on your smartphone to check the app, fitness tracker, Healthy Habit Tool, etc. that includes your SMART goals.

- **Strengthen your "NO muscle."** When you're feeling tempted by others to do something that takes you off course from your goals, have a comeback ready that's easy to remember. This will take you to newer, better places as you learn to prioritize your life and create the resources (time, money, energy, etc.) to do what's best for you. Once you're on board, you'll find you've got more resources to do what you know feels right. Eventually, these new strategies will be easier to implement and manage.

- **Plan ahead.** As the saying goes, "Failing to plan is planning to fail." So create a regular plan for how you'll build more motion into your life. Write it down so it's in black and white. Schedule the 10-Minute Body Maintenance System in your calendar just as you would a very important appointment. Make it as much a non-negotiable as your shower or morning coffee. Then put things in place that will help keep you on track.

These suggestions are just a few of many ways you can remain more committed to achieving your vision, make the Tools & Techniques convenient so you will use them, and become more consistent in your daily practices. With this foundation, you can learn how to create the habits that will support your active, pain-free lifestyle.

10

Create Habits That Support Your Active Lifestyle

"It's never too late to redefine self-control, to change long ingrained habits, and to do the work you're capable of."

—SETH GODIN

You now know how focusing on the 3Cs can support the habits you'll need to master. But how do you actually create those good habits required to support your pain-free lifestyle? Knowledge is power, and I've found it helpful to dig deeper into the psychology and biology of behavior change and habits in general. So, let's explore what habits are, how they form, and how to create new ones to support our active lifestyle.

The Truth About Habits.

Habits are learned mindsets or activities that, over time, require little to no effort by our bodies and our brains. A habit is a behavior you do without thinking; it should be more or less automatic.

In forming new habits, the simplest place to start is focusing on new behaviors or routines you actually *want to do*. If a particular new behavior or routine feels like a "should"—something you're forced to do—it probably will not become a true habit. So when you're learning how to create a new habit, don't focus on the obligation; instead, focus on the core desired feelings you intentionally want to create (defined in Part I).

Creating a new habit is the cornerstone to your success as you take action and apply everything you've been given in this guidebook. The goal is to adopt new, healthy habits that will enable you to achieve your goals. But if you don't know how to create those habits, you won't change.

One of my favorite ways to understand how habits are created comes from author Charles Duhigg in his book *The Power of Habit*. Using science-based research, Duhigg concludes that habits form through a "feedback loop." The feedback loop includes three elements:

- first, the **cue** that kickstarts thinking or acting automatically;
- then, some physical and/or emotional **routine** (something you do that may or may not be automatic);
- and finally, the **reward** that tells your brain whether it's worth remembering the next time you're facing that familiar cue. If the reward is worth remembering, then the likelihood of a habit developing goes up. In essence, habits get set as that reward gets higher or feels better.[26]

According to Duhigg: The reason the discovery of the habit loop is so important is that it reveals a basic truth: When a habit emerges, the brain stops fully participating in decision making. It stops working so hard, or diverts focus to other tasks. So unless you deliberately fight a habit —unless you find new routines—the pattern will unfold automatically.

Think about the habit loop this way: Can you identify with a midday slump and the desire to have a sugary treat? If you are not aware of the cue-routine-reward feedback loop, then the routine of an occasional midday sweet can turn into a bad habit. If we can interrupt and change this routine, however, we can create a new habit.

The same goes for the 10-Minute Body Maintenance System. I regularly work with people who have a hard time being consistent with the system and therefore have a hard time making it a habit. They are extremely committed to living pain-free; however, they struggle to make their efforts convenient (part of a *routine*) so they can be consistent and form a new habit. By making the system part of their everyday routine, it can eventually become a habit that helps them achieve their pain-free vision.

The Feedback Loop

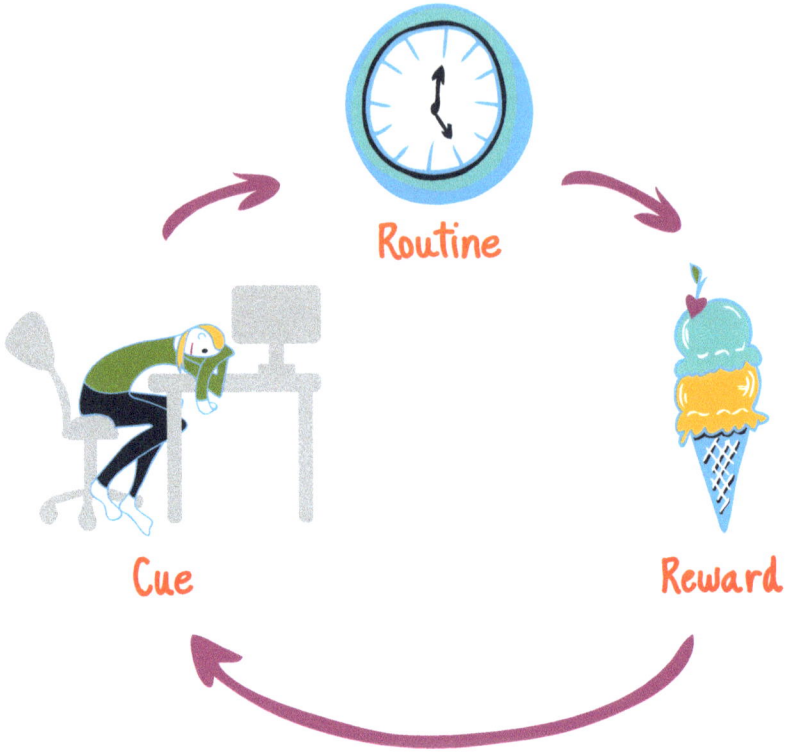

Routine

Cue

Reward

How Do I Create a New Habit?

There are a number of ways to create new habits based on the feedback loop:

1. Change the cue
2. Change the routine
3. Change the reward

First, we can *change the cue*s that trigger habits. So if you hang around negative people who trigger you to talk about negative things like your pain, try shifting your social circle to include new, positive, and forward-focused friends. I bet you will eventually talk and think more about possibility and less about pain. You can also surround yourself with other resources to reinforce your commitment—listen to podcasts while you exercise, read inspiring books, watch TED Talks when folding laundry, and start your day with gratitude practices. Adopt that more grateful mindset for each bit of progress you've made.

Second, you can change your habits by *changing the reward* you want. If you've determined that the feeling you desire (from Part I) is to feel comfortable in your own skin, then that reward becomes the key motivator for using the Tools & Techniques you learned in Part II. As you use these Tools & Techniques—and back them up with a focus on the 3Cs—you will make shifts away from the pain toward your possibility.

Third, habits are more likely to stick if you *change your routine*. If you shake up what you normally do between the cue and the reward, you'll be more likely to succeed. The key is to establish a new routine and then practice it until it becomes automatic. The more thinking you do about your routine (e.g., making excuses not to do it or questioning whether you should do it today), the more you increase the odds that you will not get the desired results. We are working toward creating automatic behaviors.

If you hang around negative people who trigger you to talk about negative things like your pain, try shifting your social circle to include new, positive, and forward-focused friends.

For example, if you leave your active workstation in an upright position, you'll come back to it the next morning with a visual, physical, and functional reminder or cue to stand. The same is true if you use an app, timer, or alarm clock as a reminder to move about, reset your posture, or take a movement break with the 10-Minute Body Maintenance System. You will feel more energized and ready to tackle your next task, thus creating momentum with each small success.

The Habit Loop

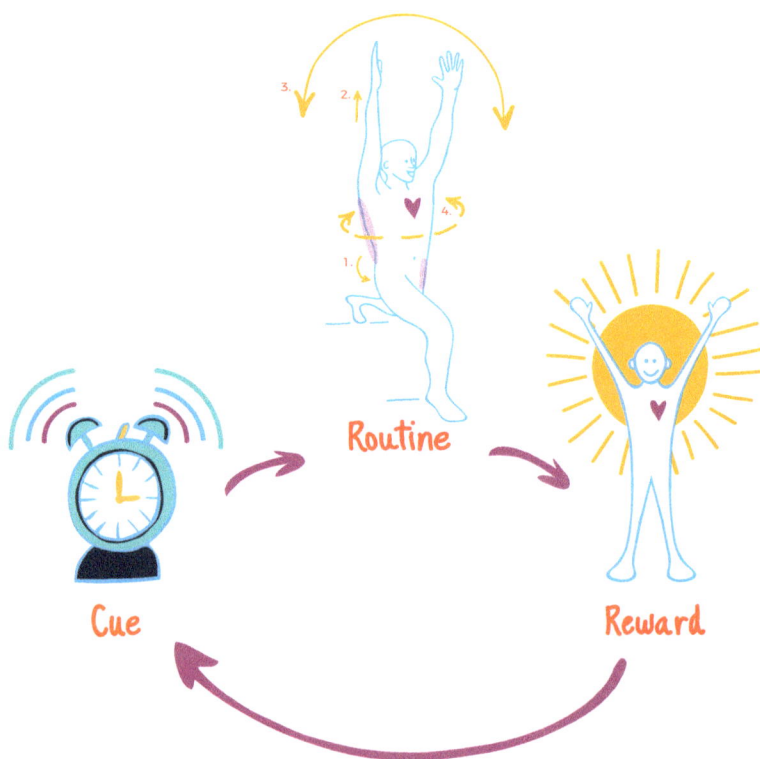

Cue → Routine → Reward

How Long Does a New Habit Take to Form?

Don't be surprised if it takes a long time to fully own these new habits. Perhaps you have heard the myth that it takes 21 days to form a habit. According to a study cited in *The British Journal of General Practice*,[27] "This myth appears to have originated from anecdotal evidence of patients who had received plastic surgery treatments and typically adjusted psychologically to their new appearance in twenty-one days." However, according to the current research, the sweet spot for forming a new habit is 66 days. I recommend giving yourself 10 weeks and understanding that forming a new habit is a process. Practice makes progress, not perfection or permanence. Some habits form quickly. Others may take a long, long time.

My experience in working with clients is that the knowledge, structure, and guidance to do the initial heavy lifting is missing when it comes to getting results and sustaining those results with healthy habits. People are reassured when I tell them that the first steps can be a lot less work if they focus on creating a new habit that actually rewards them with how they *want to feel*. Clients find that small successes build momentum, keep them motivated, and lead to more successes.

Without a doubt, people who ultimately reach their goals are those who are patient, persistent, and pace themselves as they journey through their individual process. They gain confidence with each small step taken to achieve goals that are aligned with their vision. They adopt the 3Cs and create new habits that enable them to live pain-free, energized, and confident. In this way, they can truly live their life by design.

Conclusion

"Practice makes progress.
Not perfection. Not permanence."
—HEIDI ROBERTS

This book isn't like most books where once you read it, you put it on a shelf or share it with a friend. Your journaling about your Pain & Possibility in Part I, learning the Tools & Techniques in Part II, and creating habits to achieve the Results & Outcomes in Part III are now very personal to you. They can be referred to and expanded upon time and time again as you continue on your health and wellness journey. Remember, practice makes progress. There is no such thing as perfection or permanence. Everything changes. So in light of that . . .

Keep practicing. Remain curious. Stay consistent. Live pain-free by sustaining your active lifestyle at work, at home, and at play!

As you continue to take action, welcome new knowledge that will come to you. This book is just the beginning of understanding more about yourself as a growing individual. Over time, you'll come to discover what activities support you in feeling good and how those can consistently create the feelings you desire. Practicing these strategies, techniques, and tools will support a balanced body and how *you* want to *feel*.

Let this guidebook be part of the process for transforming pain, sustaining gains, and realizing your possibility. Remember, you must stay committed if you want to experience change. Your vision of success will become real only through your personal desire, discipline, and dedication.

Keep practicing. Remain curious. Stay consistent. Live pain-free by sustaining your active lifestyle at work, at home, and at play! Take advantage of the additional resources on my website. Join in on what is called "Motion Therapy," a world in which ambitious people manage their body imbalances to live pain-free. Keep trusting in yourself. Take one step at a time as you progress on your health and wellness journey. You can do it!

Acknowledgments

Thank you, my reader, for investing in this practical guidebook to support your health and wellness journey and transform your pain into your possibility while you work!

Thank you to my teachers, coaches, and mentors who have shared their wisdom through books, courses, podcasts, interviews, phone calls, walking meetings, and adventuring.

Thank you to my all-important community of family, friends, clients, and colleagues for listening, supporting, and encouraging me on my health and wellness journey.

A special thank you to the following people for being on this wild adventure with me:

To Mom and Dad, I am the woman I am today because of both of your love, support, and encouragement. I love you!

To Eric Roberts and Teresa Roberts, I have learned from and been inspired by both of you.

To Tim, you are the love of my life. I am a better person because of the things you've taught me.

To Aunt Suz, thank you for all your love, yoga, and reminding me to follow my heart.

To Katie Roberts, Julie Rocha Buel, Christina Roth, Jennifer Stimson, and Morgan Gist MacDonald & Team for bringing your hearts and talent to this project!

To my beta readers, thank you for believing in my mission and bringing your opinions and feedback to this project. My heartfelt gratitude for each of these beautiful women with whom I have been lucky enough to be on the planet at the same time: Erica Nelson, Lisa Hill, Shelli McClung, Lianro WagenerSmith, Gabrielle McGrew, Mary Stavrou, Juliet Maris, Theresa Perry, Eileen Garvin, Kristen Anne Campbell, and Jennifer Silapie.

Appendix A:

10-MINUTE BODY MAINTENANCE EXERCISES—UPPER VS. LOWER BODY TECHNIQUES

Upper Body Techniques

Neck Stretch

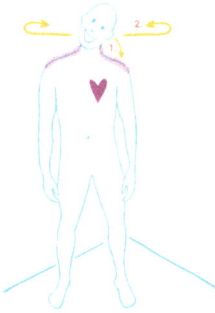

Shoulder Reset Stretch

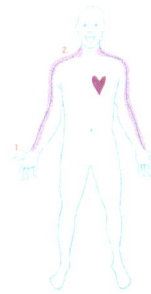

Chest Opener Stretch

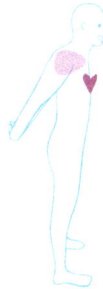

Upper Body Nerve Glide

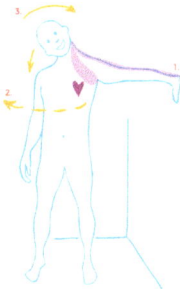

Shoulders + Mid Back Stretch

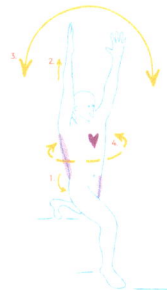

Lower Body Techniques

Piriformis Stretch

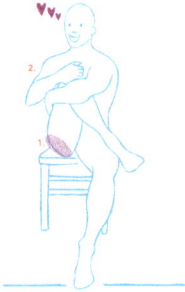

Hip + Quad Stretch

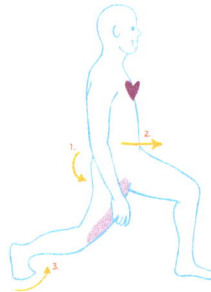

Hamstring + Low Back Stretch

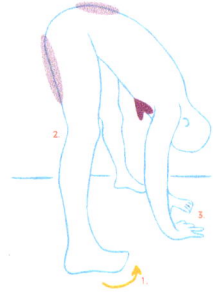

Seated Spine Stretch

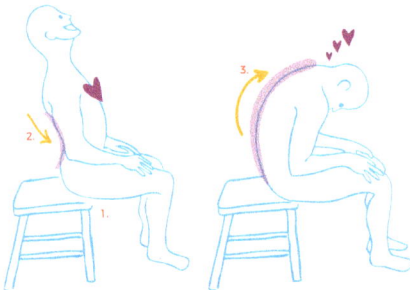

Calf + Lower Leg Stretch

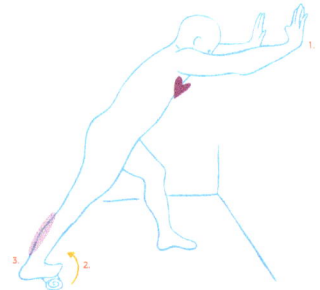

Appendix B:

HEALTHY HABIT TOOL CHART

Motion Therapy	Week 1	Week 2	Week 3	Week 4	Week 5	Week 6	Week 7	Week 8	Week 9	Week 10
Monday										
Tuesday										
Wednesday										
Thursday										
Friday										
Saturday										
Sunday										
Done on 5 days? Y or N										
How natural did it feel? ☹ 😐 🙂										

Goal: 10-Minute Body Maintenance

Notes

1. Selene Yeager, "Sitting Is the New Smoking—Even for Runners," *Runner's World*, accessed March 4, 2016, http://www.runnersworld .com/health/sitting-is-the-new-smoking-even-for-runners.

2. Gretchen Reynolds, "Get Up. Get Out. Don't Sit," *The New York Times* (blog), October 17, 2012, accessed March 4, 2016, http://well .blogs.nytimes.com/2012/10/17/get-up-get-out-dont-sit/?_r=0.

3. Karen Ravn, "Don't Just Sit There. Really," *Los Angeles Times*, May 25, 2013, accessed March 4, 2016, http://articles.latimes .com/2013/may/25/health/la-he-dont-sit-20130525.

4. Florida Atlantic University, "Sobering Statistics on Physical Activity in the U.S.," *Science Daily*, August 26, 2015, accessed April 4, 2016, https://www.sciencedaily.com /releases/2015/08/150826093015.htm.

5. "The Chronic Pain Epidemic: What's to Be Done?," interview by David Freeman, The Forum at the Harvard T.H. Chan School of Public Health, forum video, November 10, 2016, https://theforum. sph.harvard.edu/events/the-chronic-pain-epidemic/.

6. M. W. Brault, J. Hootman, C. G. Helmick, K. A. Theis, and B. S. Armour, "Prevalence and Most Common Causes of Disability Among Adults—United States, 2005," report, *MMWR Weekly* 58, no. 16 (May 1, 2009): 421–26, accessed March 4, 2016, http://www.cdc.gov/mmwr/preview/mmwrhtml/mm5816a2 .htm.

7. Centers for Disease Control Foundation, "Worker Illness and Injury Costs U.S. Employers $225.8 Billion Annually," news release, January 28, 2015, http://www.cdcfoundation.org /pr/2015/worker-illness-and-injury-costs-us-employers-225 -billion-annually.

8. Julie Corliss, "Too Much Sitting Linked to Heart Disease, Diabetes, Premature Death," *Harvard Health Blog, Harvard Health Publications of Harvard Medical School,* January 22, 2015, accessed March 4, 2016, http://www.health.harvard.edu/blog/much-sitting-linked -heart-disease-diabetes-premature-death-201501227618.

9. J. Lennert Veerman, et al., "Television Viewing Time and Reduced Life Expectancy: A Life Table Analysis," *British Journal of Sports Medicine* 46, no. 13, accessed March 4, 2016, http://bjsm.bmj .com/content/46/13/927.full.

10. N. P. Pronk, et al., "Reducing Occupational Sitting Time and Improving Worker Health: The Take-a-Stand Project, 2011," *Preventing Chronic Disease* 9:110323 (2012), October 11, 2012, accessed March 4, 2016, http://www.cdc.gov/pcd /issues/2012/11_0323.htm.

11. John Buckley, "How Standing Up in the Office Can Help You Lose Weight," *University of Chester,* January 9, 2013, accessed March 4, 2016, http://www.chester.ac.uk/node/16952.

12. Yeager, "Sitting Is the New Smoking."

13. IU Bloomington Newsroom, "Taking Short Walking Breaks Found to Reverse Negative Effects of Sitting," news release, September 8, 2014, accessed March 4, 2016, http://news.indiana.edu /releases/iu/2014/09/slow-walking-sitting-study.shtml.

14. Pronk, et al., "Reducing Occupational Sitting Time."

15. Stacy A. Clemes, et al., "Reducing Children's Classroom Sitting Time Using Sit-to-Stand Desks: Findings from Pilot Studies in UK and Australian Primary Schools," *Journal of Public Health (Oxford)* 38, no. 3 (2016): 526–33, accessed April 4, 2016, http://jpubhealth.oxfordjournals.org/contentearly/2015/06/14 /pubmed.fdv084.abstract.

16. Ergotron, "New Survey: To Sit or Stand? Almost 70% of Full Time American Workers Hate Sitting but They Do It All Day Every Day," news release, July 17, 2013, accessed March 14, 2016,

http://www.prnewswire.com/news-releases/new-survey-to-sit
-or-stand-almost-70-of-full-time-american-workers-hate-sitting
-but-they-do-it-all-day-every-day-215804771.html.

17. Corliss, "Too Much Sitting Linked to Heart Disease, Diabetes, Premature Death."

18. Kyndall L. Boyle, Josh Olinick, and Cynthia Lewis, "The Value of Blowing Up a Balloon," *North American Journal of Sports Physical Therapy* 5, no. 3 (2010): 179, accessed March 14, 2016, http://www.ncbi.nlm.nih.gov/pmc/articles/PMC2971640/.

19. Andy Puddicombe, "All It Takes Is 10 Mindful Minutes," TED video, 5:13, posted January 2013, https://www.ted.com /talks/andy_puddicombe_all_it_takes_is_10_mindful_minutes /transcript?language=en.

20. Kulinski, et al., "Association Between Cardiorespiratory Fitness and Accelerometer-Derived Physical Activity."

21. Belle Beth Cooper, "The Science of Posture: Sitting Up Straight Will Make You Happier, More Confident, and Less Risk-Adverse," *Buffer Social* (blog), *Buffer*, November 11, 2013, accessed April 2, 2016, https://blog.bufferapp.com/improve-posture-good -posture-science-happiness.

22. Peter Le and William S. Marras, "Evaluating the Low Back Biomechanics of Three Different Office Workstations: Seated, Standing, and Perching," *Journal of Applied Ergonomics*, no. 56 (2016): 170–78, https://www.ncbi.nlm.nih.govpubmed/27184325.

23. David Butler, G. Lorimer Moseley, and Sunyata, "Pacing and Graded Exposure" in *Explain Pain* (Adelaide, Australia: Noigroup Publications, 2003), 114.

24. Marie Forleo, "Why You'll Never Find Your Passion," *MarieForleo .com*, accessed March 14, 2016, https://www.marieforleo .com/2014/04/find-your-passion.

25. "John Maxwell on Leadership, Living Big, and Choosing a Life That Matters," interview by Lewis Howes, audio video, *The School*

of Greatness: The Blog of Lewis Howes, accessed March 14, 2016, http://lewishowes.com/podcast/john-maxwell/.

26. Charles Duhigg, *The Power of Habit: Why We Do What We Do in Life and Business* (New York: Random House, 2014), 19.

27. Benjamin Gardner, Phillippa Lally, and Jane Wardle, "Making Health Habitual: The Psychology of 'Habit-Formation' and General Practice," *British Journal of General Practice* 62, no. 605 (2012): 665, accessed March 14, 2016, http://www.ncbi.nlm.nih.gov/pubmed/23211256.

Glossary

Active workstation: a workspace designed to allow both aligned sitting and standing in order to optimize your body's performance. Commonly called "standing desks," "standing workstations," or "sit-stand workstations," active workstations enhance our mental, physical, and emotional health; support better digestion and overall body function; and can help lower the risk of Sitting Disease.

Aligned sitting: a technique designed to improve head-to-hip alignment and muscle engagement of the upper body; see also *aligned standing*.

Aligned standing: a technique designed to improve your standing alignment while engaging muscles of your entire body, specifically the pelvis, spine, shoulders, neck, upper back, and chin. Aligned standing assists you in moving properly as you remain active throughout the day. See also *aligned sitting*.

Alignment: the proper arrangement of all the body's muscles and bones. When all 640 muscles and 206 bones are in optimal alignment, your "system" is primed for optimal performance, and you can perform activities efficiently, effectively, and without pain or limitation. See also *posture*.

Body scan: a quick but powerful assessment tool for identifying pain in your body. Whether you're sitting still or standing still, it can help you notice what you are feeling, where you are feeling it, and how intense it is.

Cue: the first part of forming a habit according to the "feedback loop." The cue kickstarts thinking or acting automatically. See also *routine* and *reward*.

Goals: practical, attainable outcomes that you plan for and believe move you toward your vision. More than mere hopes or wishes, they are concrete stepping-stones that lead you down the path of a valued life. See also *short-term goals* and *long-term goals*.

Habit: a behavior you do without thinking; a learned mindset or activity that, over time, requires little to no effort by our bodies and our brains. See also *practice* and *routine*.

Long-term goals: goals that become your ultimate reality, or part of your life. Long-term goals may include lifelong habits such as incorporating the 10-Minute Body Maintenance System into your daily practice. See also *short-term goals*.

Lower Crossed Syndrome: muscular imbalances focused in the lower part of the body that are caused by poor posture and alignment. The source of imbalance is in opposing groups of tight muscles and weak muscles. See also *Upper Crossed Syndrome*.

Mindful breathing: proactively engaging your breathing muscles in a natural, balanced way while you breathe. Mindful breathing contributes to good alignment and enables greater mobility. It also provides the added benefit of calming the heart, mind, and body as a whole, highly integrated system; it enables greater patience for where you're at, what you notice, and what you feel. See also *mindfulness*.

Mindfulness: exercises or techniques aimed to increase awareness of the body, mind, and/or spirit and to improve focus on the task at hand. For the purposes of this book, mindfulness includes mindful breathing with the balloon breathing technique, *body scans*, and routine body work, such as the stretching exercises included in the 10-Minute Body Maintenance System. These practices ultimately help us make better choices in our journey of health and wellness. See also *mindful breathing*.

Nerve gliding: muscle stretches that help soft tissue move properly and therefore prevent related pain. Nerve gliding is aided by the body maintenance tools mentioned in this book, specifically the Stretch Out Strap and foam roller.

Posture: a snapshot of how you hold your body at any given moment. Proper posture is an outward sign that your body is accurately aligned. Posture is about what's seen, while alignment is about what's connected. See also *alignment*.

Practice: repeated exercise in or performance of an activity or skill so as to acquire and maintain proficiency in it. See also *habit* and *routine*.

Reward: the third part of forming a habit according to the "feedback loop." If your brain thinks a reward is worth remembering, then the likelihood of a habit developing increases. See also *cue* and *routine*.

Routine: something (physical and/or emotional) you do often that may or may not be automatic; the second part of forming a habit according to the "feedback loop." Healthy, consistent routines can help create good habits, such as practicing the 10-Minute Body Maintenance System every day. See also *habit* and *practice; cue* and *reward*.

Self-pacing and graded exposure: part of a step-by-step plan, described in depth in *Explain Pain*, that can boost the odds of success in accomplishing goals; steps include choosing what to do more, noting your baseline, planning your progression, accepting flare-ups, and making it your lifestyle.

Shift: a change in awareness of a sensation (e.g., relief, release, or greater mobility) that gets you closer to how you want to feel in your body. The exercises throughout this book help generate a shift toward your pain-free possibility.

Short-term goals: goals that equate to small successes and create momentum as you achieve them. Short-term goals are made based on what you want to accomplish and how you want to feel now. They support your *long-term goals* and ultimately, your *vision*.

Sitting Disease: the state of physical, mental, or emotional pain that results from having a sedentary lifestyle. The symptoms include everything from neck and back pain to depression, obesity, heart disease, and even cancer. Sitting Disease leads to acute and chronic health-care conditions and is a contributing factor to *Lower Crossed Syndrome* and *Upper Crossed Syndrome*.

SMART goals: long-term and short-term goals that are **S**pecific, **M**easurable, **A**ttainable, **R**ealistic, and **T**ime-bound. Setting goals with each of these five attributes improves your success in achieving them. See also *long-term goals* and *short-term goals*.

Soft tissue: includes tendons, ligaments, fascia, skin, synovial membranes, muscles, nerves, and blood vessels. Proper and regular movement of the soft tissue helps prevent pain.

Trigger point: a sensitive area of the body that gets so irritated that the body misinterprets the pain signal, causing the person to feel as if the pain is coming from somewhere else. The five body maintenance tools and exercises mentioned in this book can help release trigger points.

Upper Crossed Syndrome: muscular imbalances in the upper body caused by poor posture and alignment. The source of imbalance is in the opposing group of tight muscles and weak muscles. See also *Lower Crossed Syndrome*.

Vision: the big, broad goal in your life. Your vision is the exciting picture of your future, your ultimate destination. It determines why you need to do—or not do—what you're doing. Your vision should be purposely crafted to motivate and inspire you to live an energized, confident, and pain-free life. See also *goals*.

About the Authors & Illustrator

Heidi Roberts is a doctor of physical therapy and the founder of Motion Therapy. She is passionate about educating and empowering people to use movement to correct imbalances in the body, mind, and spirit so they can live pain-free. Based in Hood River, Oregon, she lives an active lifestyle, embraces lifelong learning, and pursues optimal health and wellness through regular outdoor adventures.

Katie Roberts has a passion for communications and media. Her career highlights include television reporting for ABC News, serving as an award-winning managing editor for a national bridal/wedding business magazine, and creating and managing a successful Colorado-based nonprofit. In 2006, Katie launched her own freelance writing/editing business, Write on Target! Communications, based in Hood River, Oregon.

Julie Rocha Buel is an illustrator and designer based in Hood River, Oregon, where she lives with her husband and two children. Julie is fiercely passionate about making a positive impact on the world through soulful art and intentional design. Her work is inspired by nature and the pursuit of creating a meaningful life for herself and others.

www.ingramcontent.com/pod-product-compliance
Lightning Source LLC
Chambersburg PA
CBHW060318310326
41914CB00102B/1993/J